The

5000th

Baby

Dedication

With lots of love and admiration for our baby, our families, our friends, our care providers, as well as dedicated to all those who are dealt with the cards of medical adversities, who have their own journeys, roadmaps, milestones, outcomes and reflections about the same.

DISCLOSURE

This book is based upon a true story. It is based upon the author's best recollection of events and reconstruction of the story. The names of some clinicians and hospitals have been changed to maintain anonymity, while trying to preserve the focus on depiction of the situations, perceptions and emotions, rather than finding blame. The contents of this book should not be used for any clinical decision making purposes. Patients and families are encouraged to work with and consult their physicians and care teams to help make the most appropriate decisions for their child, while taking their child's and family's unique situation in mind. Lastly, it is quite likely that the current infrastructure, facilities and practices in the hospitals mentioned in this book are currently different than the ones depicted in the book, since 14 years have elapsed since the occurrence of the events and the publication of this book.

ACKNOWLEDGEMENTS

First, I would like to thank Sheri my wife, the love of my life, and the mother of my two children, for encouraging me to write this book over the past several years. She helped shape the book's contents by providing valuable suggestions, and insights to my draft version, as it evolved into the book that you now see in print. I cannot imagine the journey without her love and support as we collectively navigated the twists and turns of the complex roadmap of surgeries, treatments and regimens for our son.

Special thanks to my parents, my aunt (referred to Mavshi in the book), my brother and sister in law, as well as Sheri's family, and our family friends (Harkamal and Dimple) who all in their own way, provided an essential and crucial infrastructure of encouragement and love that helped us in our ability to provide the best care possible for Rajan that resulted in a good outcome for him.

My heartfelt thanks go to Dr. Adrian Nedelcut and his wife Melissa Nedelcut for their encouragement and support for this book. Adrian provided lots of feedback and perspective from a reader's point of view, and I was honored to include his thoughts in the foreword. My sincere thanks go to Melissa for her painstaking attention to detail as she reviewed and edited the entire book, while providing excellent critique, feedback and suggestion to help improve readability of the book.

My special thanks got to my two special friends, colleagues and partners in improvement – Dr. Donna Claes and Dr. Jennifer Lail who were always personally there for me, especially in our most critical times of need during our child's course of care.

Words cannot express the gratitude and respect I have for the providers of medical care for our son. These are the pediatric healthcare professionals that pour their heart and soul into caring for the patient and giving information, guidance and hope to the families of patients so that they may be able to care for the patient too.

My heartfelt thanks go to Ronald McDonald Houses for providing us a home away from home when seeking treatment for Rajan that was hundreds of miles away from our home town.

A big shout out to my sons Roshan and Rajan for reading, reviewing, and providing valuable suggestions for improving the readability of the book.

FOREWORD 1

In my seven years as Assistant Vice President for Chronic Care at Cincinnati Children's Hospital Medical Center, Mr. Dahale, a very professional industrial engineer, was my colleague. He served as Senior Quality Improvement Consultant for the Division of Pediatric Nephrology, which ranked # 3 in the nation for its care for children and youth with kidney disorders. As part of the children's Nephrology team, his expertise in quality improvement methodologies and system improvements was obvious, working with doctors, nurses, medical assistants, families, data analysts and informatics specialists to improve the care and clinical outcomes for these children. What distinguished his work, though, was his earnest passion for care that centered around the child and family, and reliably applied the very best medical and surgical knowledge to help every child get better.

Gradually, as we discussed lab-work, blood pressure measurement and maintaining kidney function, my colleagues and I began to hear his own child and family's story emerging in the workplace. Only then did we understand his intensity and quest for excellence; he informed and inspired all of us who worked alongside him. The detail and precision he applied at work is mirrored in his book, "The 5000th Baby", combining his lived experience with technical expertise. Devesh recounts his own son Rajan's story of being born with a complex birth defect and their grueling journey toward survival, health and triumph, with forthright revelations of his evolution as a parent, husband and health care consumer.

Families, health professionals and anyone who has entered a health care system will relate to Devesh's accounting of both extraordinary and sub-standard care, paralyzing fear and informed reassurance, battles to pay for care and the life-saving support of family and friends for a child who never chose to be ill.

Over my 41 years as a pediatrician for kids with chronic conditions, the numbers of children like Rajan, who survive and thrive with previously life-limiting conditions, has risen dramatically. We see their families grapple daily with their child's growth, education and development, complicated by medications, equipment, procedures and the personal and financial costs of convoluted health systems.

In his work, Devesh funnels his knowledge of those challenges into his role as Director for Health Systems Engineering, driving improvements in the safety, reliability and compassion in health care delivery. In his own story's blend of science, engineering, personal fortitude and profound love, he infuses us all with hope, and the conviction that every child deserves exceptional, safe and affordable health care.

Jennifer Lail, M.D., FAAP
Former AVP of Chronic Care, James M. Anderson Center for
Health Systems Excellence and Associate Professor of
Pediatrics, Complex Care Center, Cincinnati Children's
Hospital Medical Center
Jennifer Lail, LLC, Principal Consultant, Durham, NC

PREFACE

It is my privilege and a pleasure to write these brief words as a way of preface for the book "THE 5000th BABY". The writer, Mr. Dahale, is the father of one of my dear patients. He describes in a rather vivid way, his and his wife's painful experiences in dealing with their son, born with an anorectal malformation. The reading of the book will be a revealing experience for those parents of children born with this kind of defects. The book will also provide valuable information about what to do and what not to do in similar situations. The author also describes in a candid way, the multiple adverse events that he and his wife experienced when their beloved baby went through operations and complications. All these negative experiences were aggravated by the confrontation of a complicated and inefficient, medical insurance system.

Behind all this, one can perceive a justified protest against a less than optimal medical and surgical care and a plea for a more humanized and personal medical system.

Alberto Peña, MD, FAAP, FACS, FRCS | Ponzio Family Chair for Colorectal Pediatric Surgery | Director, International Center for Colorectal Care | Children's Hospital Colorado | Professor of Surgery University of Colorado

LIGHT OUT OF THE DARKNESS

A lighthouse stands atop of a cliff. It took years to build it, and the storms have made bringing materials together and raising it difficult. It was made because the light was needed to save the lives of future crews from being shipwrecked on the reefs below. Once completed, it stands as a guide for ships to use its message to find safe passage through the worst of storms.

Our eyes and minds fleetingly glimpse at the human lighthouses around us, the libraries and depositories of knowledge, of truth derived from the experiences that others share. We pass by most, as we rush through life, some bookmarked for a future review that might never take place, whereas most go forgotten... until the inexplicable happens. Like a lighthouse that shines bright and can be seen from everywhere, the detail of Sheri and Devesh's first year of life with their son emits a message that resonates with everyone who was impacted by healthcare (or is part of healthcare) on a deep, and personal level.

What can bring more joy to a person than knowing that they will be a parent, and will be able to hold their baby for the first time? Your perception of time stops in awe of the creation of life, and your heart is filled with the beautiful blessing of seeing your child, and realizing that from then on you share a unique bond that infuses the present with happiness and gives hope for the future. As a parent you expand the universe for your children, you walk with them, and explain the world, you unfold the dimensions in which they will explore and then mold their own path. Devesh and Sheri did not enjoy such a future, as their lives were changed at the moment their son was born.

How crushing can the prospect be of losing this precious life to something that comes out of nowhere, unleashing a cascade of questions, and a plunge into an unknown world of clinical decisions that must be taken emergently? How difficult is it to trust and hope that everything will be all right, to not give up in finding a better way, to keep asking questions until you have at least one right answer? How, as a parent, can you keep calm and move forward while caring for a recovering spouse, a toddler that's at home, not understanding why his parents are away to the hospital for so long, and a new born child that is taken out of your arms, so that someone you never met can operate on them, hoping that it will help?

Whether you're a parent, clinician, or both, this book resonates with you from every page. The story portrays a clear and sobering picture, one too frequent, but rarely put on paper. It is one of patients needing answers, comfort, clear plans, and quality care. On the other side is the medical system that moves patients through one call at a time, one surgery at a time, one short answer that creates more confusion and questions at a time, or that can also bring unexpected solutions, comfort, and hope.

Sheri and Devesh's story is similar to those of many patients confronted with a medical system that is stretched thin. They reach out for anyone who can be their partner in care and take the time to provide them with answers, compassion, clear communication, and effective solutions. This is a clear picture of the parents' struggles born as a response to the system's failures and disconnect, of the patches created by parents who are doing everything they can to help their children get the care they deserve. It is also a story of how a couple's love for their child fuels their strength and determination, despite the incredible obstacles that they are confronted with.

The Dahales grab hold of any fragment of hope, and with a mind focused on finding solutions, they do what any parent would do – look for answers, find questions they should ask, look for better care. But on top of that they never, ever give up. No matter how long the marathon is, their child will be taken care of correctly and he will have a normal life. There is no other acceptable outcome.

The message of this book is a blueprint for any patient who is confronted with a similar situation, and for every clinician who can now see through the eyes of their patients. In the end, this story is one of success, like a universal truth shining from a lighthouse: that love conquers, as parents will never stop caring for their children, and clinicians will never stop caring for their patients.

Adrian Nedelcut M.D.

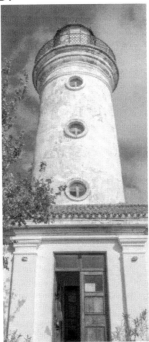

Lighthouse in Sulina, Romania.

FOREWORD 2

I first met Devesh Dahale in October 2013. I was a new faculty member within the Division of Pediatric Nephrology at Cincinnati Children's, and I was given the goal to build a care delivery system for patients with chronic kidney disease. Along with defining medical outcomes of chronic kidney disease, a major goal was to understand the patient and family perspective of managing a chronic illness such as chronic kidney disease and build support systems to help patients and families build resilience in the management of chronic illness.

This type of endeavor takes a large and diverse number of people – nurses, computer programmers, project managers. Devesh Dahale was the quality improvement manager assigned to help with the project. Over the next 5 years, I got to work alongside Devesh as he helped guide me in building this program. During this time I learned so much about Devesh and his family, and their journey with Rajan.

Throughout my time working with Devesh, I learned a lot about Devesh's son, Rajan. This book tells the story of the Dahale family, starting at the diagnosis of an anorectal malformation that was diagnosed soon after Rajan's birth. Looking at Rajan today – you see this well-adjusted teenage male who has the world in front of him. You would never know the journey it took for Rajan – as well as Devesh, Sheri, and Roshan – to be where they are today. As I read the story, I remembered many of the stories Devesh shared about the "lived experience" of chronic illness.

These stories really hit home to me. As a physician who provides medical care to children with chronic kidney disease and end stage kidney disease, I have had to look at the faces of parents like Devesh and Sheri, and explain to them that their child has a chronic illness. These conversations are never easy. But an important part of this conversation with families is providing some reassurance that things are going to be okay.

Although I provide reassurance, I know that my job is to direct the medical care. But I know that I am not the person taking this child home, and that I am not the one providing the day to day care and advocating for the best needs of their child. At this time, I offer these families an introduction to other families who have lived this experience. But not all families have this luxury. A book like this can be that support. Although this book focuses specifically on dealing with an anorectal malformation, I feel that the beauty of this book is that it can be applicable to many families dealing with chronic illness.

As a friend of the Dahale family as well as a pediatrician who provides care for children with chronic illness, this book is a great reminder to me about chronic illness from the eyes of the family. I hope you enjoy it as much as I did.

Best,

Donna J. Claes, MD BS Pharmacy

PROLOGUE

We live in a world where we are constantly bombarded with statistics. Whether it is the percentage of chance for showers coming from the daily forecast or the odds of winning the power ball, we are influenced, lured and almost always affected by probabilities and randomness all the time. Yet, we carry with ourselves the knowledge and confidence that our drive to and from work, and the bite that we grabbed at the café or a fast food restaurant will be just fine despite the low yet inherent risks of car crashes and food poisoning. In short, we live our lives with a risk adjustment meter of sorts that helps us make choices in a predictable unpredictable world.

When you chose to go on a roller coaster, or zip lining or sky diving, you can feel a palpable sense of the risk meter reflected in your resting heart rate and rate of breathing. When rare events occur, we are generally interested in two aspects – their cause and their frequency of occurrence. Frequency of occurrence is simply a reflection of our ability to count and document such events reliably, but when it comes to assigning cause, things become much trickier. Rare events are often multi-factorial in nature and history is testimony to our inability to assess the correct cause(s). Therefore we coined words such as chance, probability of occurrence, idiopathic, and randomness.

Depending upon our ability to determine the correct cause accurately (assuming we are measuring its frequency accurately), we refer to causes as idiopathic (absence of confirmed cause) and events as random (absence of specific pattern). In the field of medicine (often referred to as the youngest science), there is more to be yet learned than what has been discovered thus far, despite the rapid advances in recent decades. Birth defects is one such mysterious and grey area of science that has fascinated many a scientists.

As of writing of this book, roughly 60% of all known birth defects have an assignable cause. To put this in perspective, 40% of babies born with birth defects come as a surprise to parents, clinicians and scientists alike. However, in most of the 60% of known birth defect babies, the knowledge of the cause may still come as a surprise to the parents, even though it is known to science. This discrepancy is due to psychosocial and economic reasons. As expecting parents, we generally don't pay attention to such things, much like you don't research flight calamities before boarding an airplane or check the latest statistics on cruise ship disasters before embarking on a week-long cruise. Moreover, you are even less likely to think about such possibilities, if your previous experience with such an activity has been successful.

After our first son was born as a healthy baby (minus the slight fever at birth that resulted in him being monitored for 48 hours), we had no reason to think that the next generally healthy pregnancy (accompanied by unremarkable wellness tests and exams throughout) would result in any surprises. Surprises such as anorectal malformations (defects that fall under a spectrum of inadequate / improper development of the rectum and anus of the baby while in the fetus) happen to be part of the large variety of birth defects with an unassignable cause. Anorectal malformations occur at a frequency of <u>one in 5000 babies </u>born.

The 5000th Baby is the story of one such baby who was born with this type of defect after 4999 babies without this problem. No wonder, news of birth defects is received by parents with disbelief followed by "why me / why us?" types of questions, followed by self-blame.

This is also a story of chance in the form of coincidences reflected in the circumstantial and environmental factors that play an equally important role in the outcome of such babies in the long term. Where you are born, the existence, and access to knowledge of diagnostic and treatment methods, all play a critical role in the probability of success after you have taken the physiologic, genetic and pathologic reasons out of the equation.

This book provides you with a detailed account of the first year of the life of such a baby as viewed through the lens of the family. After having accounted for the above mentioned factors, you then encounter the plethora of variation in real life decision making, variation in skills and competencies in care providers and several known and unknown success factors of care delivery from care providers and care takers. So, without further ado, we invite you to read about the story of the 5000th baby and travel the journey, and experience the milestones across the roadmap of the baby born with an anorectal malformation. While the book addresses a specific category of anorectal malformation within the spectrum of such malformations, we hope that all patients and families of anorectal malformations as well as other birth defects, and at large those who encounter chronic disease in a pediatric or adult setting (patients, families and care providers alike), will find the events and stories in this book relevant, meaningful and thought provoking.

Devesh Dahale

TABLE OF CONTENTS

Children are a gift from the Lord; they are a reward from Him.
-Psalm 127:3

Blessed is the human birth; even the dwellers in heaven desire this birth; for true knowledge and pure love may be attained only by a human being.
-The Bhagvad Gita

CHAPTER 1: ANTICIPATION OF NEW LIFE

It was a cloudy and cold Thursday afternoon in Michigan. I looked at my watch and realized this familiar feeling of how time seemed to pass a different rate in the afternoon than it does in the morning, especially on a day when you want to get out of the office early. The "To do" list on this day was a lot more defined in the morning than it had been on any other typical day in a while. The morning went by faster than I had expected. My list involved completing as many things as I could, and then discussing the status of unfinished items with my coworkers and my boss before I left work in the afternoon. I was particularly eager to get home early that day.

As Murphy's law would have it, the same coworkers who would occasionally "hang out" in my office in the afternoons discussing a wide variety of topics such as prices of gasoline – to globalization of the industrial supplier base and similar topics (that we as a group of close knit engineers didn't realistically speaking, have much of an impact on), were suddenly difficult to locate on this afternoon. I paged them and reminded them that I was supposed to be leaving early that day and they were to stop by my office for my status updates.

After I had successfully managed to complete this rather difficult task, I told them that I was going to be taking that Friday and the following week off. My friends were aware that we were expecting our second child and they teased me – the nervous and anxious dad that I was while I continued to wrap up things and scratch off the items off my list which was already making me tired. "See you guys in about 10 days" I told my friends, and they wished me good luck as I grabbed my bag and my coat and turned off my desk computer and lights.

I had promised my wife- Sheri that I would be getting milk, bread and other such perishable essentials to last for the next few days. My maternal aunt (affectionately called "Mavshi" – a translation of the English word aunt in my native language of Marathi) had come to stay with us to help us out with the pregnancy and take care of our older son - Roshan who was going to turn three years old in a couple of months. As I walked through the mile long walkway that led to the rather large parking lot, I kept trying to remind myself of all the things I needed to do and try to block off work related things that seemed to keep popping into my mind.

As I got to the end of the walkway, I gave the familiar "nod" to the security officer at the booth and paced down the stairs with the same exact stepping that I used on those steps for the last two and a half years. I enjoyed the last whiff of warm air emitted by the radiant heaters before I stepped out into the cold windy parking lot. I looked at the parking lot and walked toward my car, which was parked in the same aisle and facing the same direction as it did each work day.

I was not much of a variety guy but rather believed in studying the intricacies of differences that were much harder to spot given that they were being extricated from events or activities that are intended to be performed the same way each time. For example, I took the same route back and forth to work, I listened to the same radio station on the way to work each day and listened to the same CD on the way back home, until I got sick of the CD or the radio station and then I would switch to a different station or CD and then would maintain consistency in that for another several months.

As I looked at the large parking lot that was less than half filled, I remembered the occasions when several veterans who worked in the shop would say "This entire parking lot used to be full twenty years ago... since then this place is gone down the tubes!" By some stroke of genius, I actually remembered to go to the grocery store, and it still took me two phone calls to Sheri and thirty five minutes just to get five simple items that I couldn't seem to easily locate. "When I go with mama, she takes only a few minutes to do the shopping in the store; she knows where things are"... my two year old son would always tell me. (In my defense, my grocery shopping skills suck! I must be probably the only person in the world who successfully manages to forget an item even when it is written on a list I carry with myself!)

When I got home it had gotten dark, and the mist was making the cool breeze feel even more chilling. As I walked into the house, I tried to anticipate how different life would be with two kids in the house, instead of one. I gave my son a big hug like I always did when I got home and a little kiss to my lovely wife who was going to get a lot of weight off her belly the next day. Although it was our second child, the day before the birth of the baby is just always full of anxiety. Our first son's birth (Roshan) was through a C-section, which led to the planned date for the delivery of our second baby (which was going to be another C-section). Roshan was born on a Friday early morning. Our second son's planned arrival time to this earth was in the afternoon - also on a Friday. I could barely sleep that night, and I can only imagine how much more nervous Sheri must have been throughout the night.

Friday morning came and went, as if it didn't exist at all. We went to get checked into the same hospital where Roshan was born, so the procedures and the environment were already familiar to us.

But what was about to happen next, was going to knock the wind out of me. I had seen my share of mishaps, project failures, and other such normal equally probably unfavorable outcome of events in my life, but NOTHING could have prepared me to face what I was about to encounter!

Our lives were going to be deeply affected in more ways than I could have ever imagined…

CHAPTER 2: JOY AND SHOCK

What is the miracle of life? What goes through the minds of parents before a child is born? Sometimes, it feels like our modern day lifestyles don't allow us to even take a minute to just sit back and wonder about the miraculous phenomenon of life being created. When we think about pregnancy and childbirth, we end up focusing on which hospital will the baby be delivered in, is the location going to impact the insurance coverage, and many such important but unappealing issues that somehow seem to take away a portion of the pure joy that is meant to be experienced.

As we got to the hospital, Dr. K, the OBGYN surgeon who had also delivered our first baby, gave us a quick but sincere smile and said that she was going to go in the operating room. She said she would have someone call me at the appropriate time to come into the operating room. The image of me holding Sheri's hand as she lay on the gurney just before going into the operating room flashed before my eyes for a moment, and the whole experience almost seemed like "Déjà vu".

So many things just seemed to be so similar to our first born son's experience, that I almost couldn't tell if I was living the same life from three years ago all over again. I got prepped with the scrubs and went back to sit in the chair in the hallway right outside the operating room. I was trying to not let anxiety get the better of me and took deep breaths every so often to help me relax. Soon enough, a nurse stepped out of the operating room and signaled me to come in.

While I continued my battle with anxiety on the inside, I took another deep breath and said to myself "It's time!", and said a quick prayer in my native language in my head before walking into the delivery room. Soft music was playing in the background, and there lay Sheri surrounded by what I call as this group of "Agents of facilitation of new individual life" and the key here is "individual". It's going to be life outside of the womb. It's like turning on the ignition to fire up all operating systems independently - starting with taking the first breath of air in the free outside world.

The nurse told me to sit by the side of Sheri's head and had a partition with a curtain that isolated a major portion of the other side of Sheri's body where the surgeon and her assistants were working hard on getting the baby out. Sheri's face looked very pale and I held her hand which felt cold to the touch. I assured her that everything was going to be alright and that the baby should be here very soon. In the background was the noise of the electronic beeps, the soft music that continued playing along with a soft humming of the middle-aged anesthesiologist who stood beside me watching and monitoring the condition of Sheri.

He seemed very relaxed and looked like the kind of guy to whom this was very routine work. It's hard to imagine that the same set of events happening in that operating room were being viewed in such a wide spectrum of level of significance to the different people in the room. Who knows – there might be a rookie nurse or a resident in learning who is going to be involved in hundreds of such procedures in the future, but will always remember this one simply because it was their FIRST! To other members of the "Agents of facilitation of new life", it's probably just another entry into the statistic of their professional careers. To the parents – this is one of their most important focal points of their lives!

I think giving birth to or being there at the moment of the birth of one's own child is undoubtedly one of the most intensely powerful moments of life. It made me appreciate the feelings that my parents must have experienced when I was born. I felt like I wasn't doing as good of a job comforting Sheri, because my mind was so inundated with thoughts and emotions that it was hard to talk at the same time and so I hoped that she was receiving the communication from my mind through my touch.

The baby was breach and the surgeon had to work harder to get him out. After the short time period of about forty five minutes (that seemed to last an eternity), the magical moment in time finally arrived. The surgeon extracted the baby and cut the cord, thus enabling the baby to let out his first cry. Life had begun for this little bundle of joy. I stood and watched the surgeon hand over the baby to the nurse who carried him to a nearby crib to clean him up and perform the physical checkup. Sheri hadn't seen him yet and, with tears in her eyes, asked me what he looked like, to which I replied that he looked just as beautiful as he sounded.

I walked up to the physical checkup station in the room. I was reminded of my first son (Roshan's) birth when they had told me that he was born with a slight fever which wasn't something to be too concerned about, but I do remember him being in the NICU (Neonatal Intensive Care Unit) for observation. But, Roshan had come out of that just fine without any problems what so ever. Being a C-section baby, I thought our younger son could possibly go through that again, but having experienced the 2 day NICU stay where they had him on I.V for a few hours was not too terrible. I waited patiently and watched our new born son intently while they continued their checkup and the surgeon continued with taking care of Sheri.

Then the doctor who examined our baby came up to me and said "Sir, there is a problem we need to talk to you about."

CHAPTER 3: INTRO. TO NICU

The first thought that came to my mind was that the doctor was going to tell me something similar to what I was told when Roshan was born - which was no big deal at all. But, she went on to say that upon physical examination they found that the baby was born with a birth defect. The words "birth defect" sent shivers up my spine and my brain and my whole body was in a state of shock. As the doctor went on to explain what she had found, I am not sure if I truly comprehended anything of what she was saying at all.

"There is no anal opening in the baby, it needs to be investigated further and the pediatric surgeon will be able to perform a better diagnosis on the severity of the condition" the doctor explained further.

"But... how come....I mean what could this mean?" I stuttered still shaking. "Sir, it is hard for me to guess, but it could just be that there is a thin layer of skin covering up the opening" she continued, and my mind jumped and grabbed onto that possibility.

It was almost like I didn't even want to hear about any other possibilities. If things were to have gone bad, this was as bad as I wanted it to be – no worse. "Something like that, the voice continued, will still require the attention of the pediatric surgeon and if it's any other diagnosis, it is he who will be able to tell you more" she muttered and made a gesture which implied that she had to get going and also, that the baby had to be moved to the NICU quickly.

Sheri quickly sensed that something was amiss and asked me "What's wrong? Is the baby OK?" I didn't know how to reply to that question. The doctor promptly came to my aid and announced "We need to take the baby to the NICU and let the pediatric surgeon make a proper diagnosis of the condition rather than us trying to guess. What I can tell you is that from past experience there have been some babies that were born with differing degrees of severity of this problem. In summary, it's not an unknown problem and is not life-threatening".

The words felt like knives being stabbed into me. Sheri still had the tears of joy from just a few minutes ago. Those tears had not had a chance to be wiped or dried, when the two of us heard this shocking unbelievable news. How can such good and bad news come at the same time? It seemed impossible. It seemed like something that would happen on a TV series like E.R. Sheri wanted me to follow the baby to the NICU and make sure the baby was going to be OK. The time for making choices had arrived. The feeling of things being out of your control had just begun.

There's something about the environment in the hospital which makes you feel very insecure, unconfident and kind of helpless in a sense. Whatever be the reason you're in the hospital for, you're always praying that that doctors and nurses are available, that hopefully everything from diagnosis to treatment and recovery goes well, and that no matter what kind of reputation the hospital has, you hope that LUCK is on your side. I always wondered why it was like that. Shouldn't you feel a lot more confident in the outcome, given that there have been significant enough advancements in medical technology, treatment methods and hospital management systems?

Then I realized that it really didn't matter how much hospitals or treatment methods improved. We would still feel the same way and the reason lies in what is at stake. We're talking about human beings not functioning properly when we go to the hospital. It's different from when you take your car into a garage to get it fixed. Sheri had a quick look at the baby before he was whisked away to the NICU. The surgeon continued looking after Sheri, while I followed the baby to the NICU. As I walked with the nurse and a couple other people, I kept looking at our baby. "How could this beautiful looking baby have anything possibly wrong with him? I just hope this is all a big mistake" I spoke to myself. We took the elevator and soon reached the NICU.

The appearance of the NICU had drastically changed since I had been there the last time - which was three years ago. They had remodeled it and the portion of the room which had a glass window from which visitors other than parents could view the baby at times, was now gone. Now there was a locked door which would open only to the staff and parents of babies that were in there. I walked in, still unsure of what to expect.

They placed the baby in an incubator and within an hour of being born, he already had an I.V line hooked up to his arm. The NICU seemed quite full, yet quiet with the occasional sound of alarms going off on the monitors that recorded hart rate, breathing patterns and oxygen levels. From experience, I had known that the alarms sounded mostly because the leads that were supposed to monitor the required conditions would get loose or move over time and hence not feed signal to the system.

Most of the babies in the NICU were premature babies which made our baby stand out as the biggest baby in the entire unit (weighing in at 8 lbs. and 11 oz.). Before our second son was born, Sheri and I had several spirited discussions on the name of our "soon to arrive" baby boy. I was keen on naming our children with Indian names since I believed that the name could be the one long lasting opportunity of upholding the Indian culture and tradition, as he would live a life in a country far away from my ancestry.

Sheri had agreed with this decision as long as we picked a name we would both like – and thus came about the name "Rajan" – meaning "King" in many Indian languages. I stood by the side of our new born son – Rajan. I watched him intently. His whole body was wrapped snug in the hospital blanket except for his head and his one arm that had the I.V. line connected to it. Although hospitals are supposed to be impervious to the time of the day or day of the week, I felt the distinct effect of a Friday afternoon in the general atmosphere.

I waited patiently to find out what the next course of action was going to be. I asked the nurse when the surgeon was going to come and she replied that she wasn't sure exactly what time he would show up, but that he was going to go on his evening rounds to see all patients before he left for the day. I looked at the clock on the wall and it was a minute before 4:00 pm. All visitors got kicked out at certain times of the day such as shift change, lunch break and so on.

It was shift change - a time when they did some clean up and briefed the next shift about the status of the current patients. As I walked out of the NICU, I realized that I was being paged by Mavshi who, along with other members of my immediate family, were anxiously waiting to hear about the mother and the baby. Given that we had shared one mobile phone in the family, my pager happened to be the most reliable method for getting a hold of me.

Picture of Rajan on his first day of life.

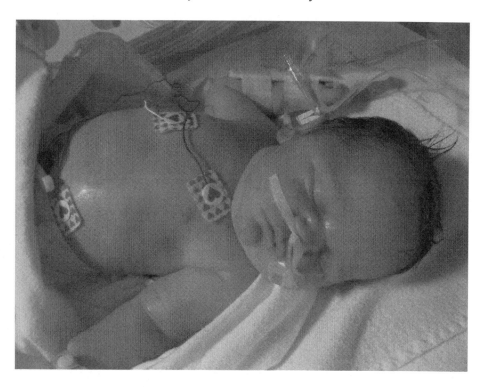

CHAPTER 4: THE DIAGNOSIS

It had been more than two hours since our son was born, and there was this strange mixture of emotions within me. I wanted to be happy that our son had just been born, but at the same time my mind was consumed with an insurmountable amount of worry and uncertainty. Although I was hoping against it, I had this feeling that something was going to go seriously wrong and it was making me sick. I also realized that I had to inform my family. I had imagined myself announcing the birth of our child to the world with lots of excitement and this unexpected situation had me very perplexed and worried. I hate to be in a position where I have to explain a situation that I am not sure about – like this one.

What should I say? That everything is alright? – That everything will be alright? Or that there is a problem with the baby but we don't know how serious it is yet? Actually, as harsh as it may have sounded, that was the truth. I was wishing for the best possible outcome and hoping for the least amount of complication, knowing that there was a complication. It couldn't pacify my mind not knowing what the actual condition was. I reached for my cell phone and made the call to Mavshi who was at home.

I could barely talk. I somehow communicated to her that things were not 100% alright, but it would take some more time to know what the real situation was, and that everyone needed to bear with the wait. I did not have the nerve or the mood to talk to my parents yet. I knew that I would break down while trying to explain the situation to my parents and that would not be a good thing at this time. I had to stay strong and be patient. I asked Mavshi to call my parents and to tell them that the baby was here and that he needed to undergo some tests and checks. I didn't want them to get worried about anything yet.

My parents were with us when our first son was born, but now they were in India, as my mom had undergone two unexpected serious back surgeries a few months prior, and had yet not fully recovered. It had been a rough year for all of us, and my mom was a little depressed and frustrated with the whole surgery ordeal. Mavshi had gladly volunteered to come and help us out. God bless her soul – I had no idea how I could have managed without her help. Mavshi made the phone calls to my parents in India and to my brother who lives in the U.K. My brother and sister-in law immediately called me back on my cell phone and tried to instill some calm in me.

I then went to check on Sheri. By the time I got back, Sheri was moved back to the general room. As I entered the room, there was silence. She was under heavy pain-relief medication and was in deep sleep. I sat in the chair by her bedside and tried to reflect on the events of the day thus far. Everything just seemed blurry and things just didn't seem to make sense, at least not yet. There were too many unanswered questions in my mind. I let Sheri rest while my mind raced at a million thoughts a minute. I waited for the hour to pass and as soon as it was 5:00 pm, I rushed upstairs to the NICU.

It looked like things had not changed much in the past hour other than the new crew that had taken over for the shift. I sat next to our baby and waited to see the nurse assigned to our baby so I could ask her what the latest status. A young looking nurse walked up to his bed and introduced herself explaining that she was going to be taking care of him for the shift.

She went on to say that the surgeon had already made rounds during the last hour and had evaluated the initial condition of the baby. I was shocked and a bit irritated to hear that. I told her that I wanted to be present when he did that and that I wanted to know more information from him. She then went on to explain that the surgeon had ordered some X-rays and ultrasounds to be performed and that he was going to be reviewing them before he left and also that he had setup a meeting time with me after he viewed the results of the tests the same evening.

Knowing that I would be speaking to the surgeon that evening, put my mind at ease for the moment. At least I was going to get a chance to ask questions and try to get a better understanding of the situation. Every now and then our little baby would let out small cries of discomfort and then go back to sleep. I waited by his bedside. The X-ray crew came by, positioned the baby appropriately to get abdominal x-rays, then left. After another half hour or so, the ultrasound team stopped by, analyzed the patient, and collected their information.

Hospitals tend to have their own pace of work, and while each parent in there might think their child needs the most urgent attention, all patients need to get appropriate attention. But, that concept is too hard for a worried parent to understand or appreciate. Finally the nurse came up to me and informed me that the surgeon was ready to talk to me in the adjoining conference room. This was going to be the moment of truth. I walked in there with my fingers crossed. The surgeon was sitting by the table along with a young looking guy. The surgeon greeted me and introduced himself and the young man who was an intern. He asked me about my work and about where I was from originally, I could tell that he was trying to make me feel a bit relaxed or comfortable before he broke the news to me. He then went on to explain the condition of our son.

The words "Birth Defect" now actually sank into me. It was much too real. He said that our son was born with something called "Imperforate anus" meaning that he did not have an anal opening, and additionally the position of the rectum was quite "high" - meaning that he is going to have to undergo a series of surgeries, the first of which needed to be performed pretty quickly. "What does this mean for how his future life is going to be?" I asked. "We need to take things one at a time" replied the surgeon. The first priority is to create a temporary bypass from within his colon by means of a "colostomy".

I was hearing a lot of these medical terms for the first time in my life. He said that the baby was in stable condition at the moment, and that they would be watching him closely until the surgery was performed. The surgeon said that normally, for this type of condition, the surgery is performed 24 hours after the baby is born. However he had the weekend off and, since the baby was in stable condition, he should be alright to be operated on the coming Monday. All this information was coming to me at a rate that I could barely deal with.

This is what I interpreted: The recommended course of action was to operate 24 hours after birth, but that if he was operated after 3 days, it would not have a negative impact as long as the baby did not get into a serious condition before then. The surgeon did assure me that if the baby's condition were to get serious enough before Monday, then he would come in on the weekend and do an emergency operation.

He asked me how I was taking all this in. I didn't know how to respond to him. He then asked me if I had any questions and I replied that I did not at this time. I replied stating that I would explain the situation the best I could, to Sheri and that we would make a list of our questions and ask them before the surgery on Monday. He told me to try not to worry too much about it and that things were going to be alright.

As we all got up ready to leave the conference room, he placed his hand over my shoulder momentarily and said "Think of it this way... your son's life over the next few years is going to be kind of a bumpy ride ... like driving on the pothole ridden roads of Michigan, but he has a pretty good chance of being just fine after that."

CHAPTER 5: IN DENIAL

I walked out of the conference room and went back to look at our little one. I looked outside the window and noticed that it was dark. The day had just flown by and while anxiety and worry were running alongside of my blood through my whole body, I was beginning to feel fatigue setting in. I looked at our son sleeping still his little body expanding and contracting with every breath he took. He looked like a little angel. Adrenalin was still pumping through my veins and I solemnly swore that I would do any and everything possible to correct the problem he has.

I blew him a kiss and transferred it gently to his forehead. I wished him goodnight and told him I loved him and proceeded to walk out of the NICU. As I got into the elevator, I wondered about how I would break the news to Sheri. There was no good way to convey this. I knew she was going to be upset and highly worried when she would hear the news. I opened the door and quietly walked into her room, not knowing if she was sleeping or not. As soon as I walked in, she opened her eyes that were still very weary from the morphine. Her voice sounded parched as she asked "How is the baby?" I explained everything I knew, and the way I understood it, to her the best I could.

Her eyes welled up with tears and I tried to console her while trying not to breakdown, myself. I told her that our son was a precious gift from God and that our love for him and his strong fighting spirit was going to get us all through this. Love, spirit, perseverance and faith from that point onward started carrying a special meaning and significance that only we would truly understand and appreciate. I thought about my other on Roshan, as he was still young enough where he was accustomed to going to sleep right by his daddy.

I had skipped lunch and now it was too late to even eat at the cafeteria that was now closed. I called Mavshi and told her that I was coming home for a while and that I would eat something real quick at home, get Roshan to bed and then come back to the hospital. I told Sheri to rest and assured her that I would be right back. As soon as I reached home, I gave a big hug to my son - Roshan. Mavshi was eager to know more about the status of Rajan and I could tell that she had not eaten lunch or dinner like me and was just consumed with worry. She had a light meal prepared for us and had fed Roshan at his regular dinner time.

I told her an abridged version of the entire situation and Mavshi told me that she and my parents have always prayed to God and that they will continue to do so and the power of prayer with everything else would get us through this difficult time. I ate dinner quickly and then laid down in bed with my son, trying to get him to sleep. I looked at Roshan and thought "How could our younger son have a major birth defect when our other son is perfectly normal and healthy?"

An endless series of questions beginning with "Why" and "How" went through my mind. The birth defect came as a surprise to everyone. There was no indication of anything wrong during the pregnancy, no indications of any abnormality in the ultrasounds, nothing that would suggest that the baby was likely to have a birth defect. These questions naturally became a part of the list of questions that we were going to ask the surgeon. I heard the steady breathing pattern from Roshan and realized that he had fallen asleep. I slowly got out of the sheets and covered him up and tucked the blankets around him and gave him a gentle kiss and whispered "Goodnight" in his ear and went to get my stuff to head back to the hospital.

I remembered that Sheri had asked for her special pillow from home and I grabbed it along with some other things that made her feel more comfortable. In this particular situation, I knew that there was nothing that would put her or my mind at ease other than our son getting through this whole ordeal alive and coming out of this in a healthy manner.

The first major event in his life was going to be the colostomy surgery. I drove back to the hospital thinking about what the surgery is going to be like, what the severity of the surgery was and what we should expect after the surgery is performed. These questions automatically appended to this mental list of questions for the surgeon that I was forming. I soon realized that I had to make sure I put down all the questions on paper so that I won't forget them.

I arrived back at the hospital and felt the exhaustion catching up with me as I walked up to Sheri's room. As I entered the room, I saw her sleeping. She was still under the influence of morphine for pain relief and rest. There was silence in the room. I opened up the chair to convert it into a bed and changed into pajamas that I had brought with me. I gently touched Sheri's hand to wish her goodnight without trying to wake her up.

As I laid back on the chair bed I realized that we had a long battle with adversity ahead of us.

As soon as I woke up the next day, I went to see our baby. I asked the nurse how he was doing and she replied that he did pretty well the previous night. After finding out that he was doing ok, I went back home to check on Roshan and Mavshi. I talked to Mavshi and Roshan for a little while and went to the basement to look up some information on the internet. I checked several medical information sites including webmd.com and others, and looked up all the search results I got in response to the keywords "imperforate anus".

A couple of articles seemed like they had plenty of information about the condition, the diagnosis and treatment and after-care. At this point of time, I was looking up more stuff that I could actually read and understand. I printed out two articles and a whole bunch of miscellaneous pages with brief information about the condition.

After a quick shower, I grabbed the print outs and rushed to the hospital. Sometimes, our brains are so preoccupied with worry that it is actually amazing that we can function at all - such as drive the car, walk, talk etc. when all that I could think of and wonder about was how my son was going to make it. Along with adversity comes the natural ability to deal with and fight with adversity. It is the essence of all life forms. The outcome of the struggle is uncertain, but the struggle itself is almost invariably inevitable.

My biggest and hardest battle however, was against the train of negative thoughts which originated from the "What ifs". What if he doesn't make it through surgery? What if the outcome of the surgery is not as expected? What if the surgeon makes a mistake? What if this hospital does not have the required resources for what my son needs? Every time I tried to block a What-if scenario from taking roots in my mind, another would pop up. I just realized that I had not smiled for thirty six hours – it was hard to even visualize how my face looked like especially since I have a generally cheerful and upbeat personality and approach toward life. At this time, there was absolutely no room for any cheer in my heart or mind. It felt as if anger, frustration and anxiety were like the heaviest pieces of traction weights hanging from every part of my body.

Another day passed by, and I continued to exist in this strange mix of adrenaline and depressive anxiety. Later that afternoon, we were getting nervous and anxious about what the next day was going to bring. We sat there patiently waiting for some updates. I had already been to the NICU and it was shift change time again.

I suddenly remembered about the papers I had printed the previous night. I took them out of the manila folder and began to read. I felt the tension mount as I continued to read – I knew that I had to prepare myself to read the contents. It was not the first time that I had read up on medical conditions – but this time it was different – it was too real and too close to home –it was about the fate of our new born child.

Roshan who came to visit and see his baby brother.

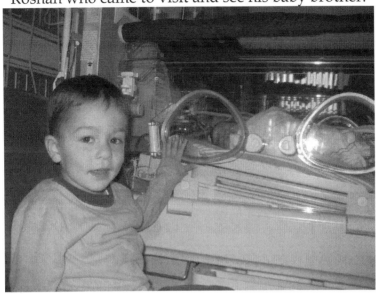

Mavshi comes to visit Rajan

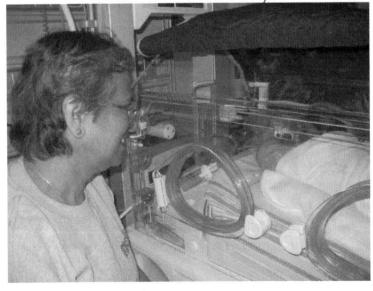

CHAPTER 6: COMING TO TERMS

It must have been about 2:00 pm. Sheri was still in a strange half awake and half asleep stage. I held her hand and she asked me if I had found out more about Rajan's condition. I told her that the hospital physician was going to stop by our room to give us an update and more information. It was a Saturday and I was expecting a resident or a junior attending doctor to be at the hospital at that time (weekend). Our minds were flooded with thoughts of uncertainty and anguish and we both drifted into a nap which was quickly interrupted with a knock on the door.

We both woke up and I instinctively stood up from my chair. Standing up as opposed to sitting down seems to convey the message that we are more attentive. It's like when you're driving and looking for a certain street or following the map, you tend to turn down the radio or music as if listening to the radio is partly occupying your attention and that you need to focus your attention on the directions.

In walked one of the residents. He didn't appear confident, but again in his defense, he was there to learn. He referred to his notes and told us that our baby was still "stable" and that they were waiting for Dr. G (the main pediatric surgeon) to perform his surgery which was most likely going to happen on Monday.

We asked him what the appropriate timing for surgery was, and he remarked stating that it is normally done 24 hours after the baby is born; however it could be done later provided the baby was still in the "stable" condition. I was hearing the word "stable" way too many times for my comfort. It just felt odd… something didn't seem right. I asked him again – "Medically speaking, when is the surgery recommended to be performed?"

He continued to give me a "beat around the bush" answer. Finally he continued "Dr. G is not available this weekend to perform the surgery and your baby is stable right now. We are monitoring him continuously and if that situation changes, we will call Dr. G and perform an emergency surgery, else your baby will be scheduled for surgery sometime on Monday."

All this talk was making us really uncomfortable and did not give us much confidence in the way Rajan's case was being handled. "What if we didn't want to wait until Monday?" I asked, to which he replied "Well, we could always look for an existing resident in surgery and see if he could do the surgery, but of course he would not be much experienced in performing such a surgery..." After he uttered those words, I was about to grab this guy by the throat and beat the crap out of him for the ridiculous responses he was giving to questions that I was asking.

But, I kept my calm and spoke in an irritated tone "You think I would want to put my child's life in the hands of a resident surgeon who does not have experience with this type of surgery?" He realized that I was upset by what he had said and then rephrased his statement and tried to reassure us that our baby would be OK and taken care of. I was starting to lose my confidence in this hospital and its services very rapidly. We ended the conversation saying that we wanted to speak to the main pediatric surgeon (Dr. G) as soon as possible and that we only requested and expected the resident to convey this message to the hospital staff and contact Dr. G.

I went back to see Rajan at the NICU later that evening. As I washed and scrubbed my hands in the sink at the entrance, I started thinking about how many times I would be doing this ritual – probably many more times than the last time when Roshan was born – he was in the NICU for just the weekend and was held there just to be monitored. But this time, I knew that the NICU stay for Rajan was going to be significantly longer.

As I walked through the aisle and through the door, I realized that the layout of the place had also changed significantly from what it was three years ago. I walked past several beds with tiny babies. Each little unit consisted of the baby bed, several monitors, equipment for IV deliveries and two chairs (a regular wooden chair and a rocking chair). I finally reached the place where Rajan was located. There he lay – still inside the incubator. He had an IV line running through his left arm and a whole bunch of leads connected across his chest and abdomen. I wanted to hold him in my arms so bad – but couldn't. The only place I could reach him was through two little windows located on the sides of the incubator. I asked a nearby nurse if I could open one so I could touch my baby. She replied that it was OK to do so and I opened the window and slowly reached my hand inside.

I decided to touch his right arm that was free from the IV connection. It was like a magical touch and it sent shivers through my body and instantly brought a tear to my eyes. I wondered what was going on inside his brain, inside his body and whether he would ever know how worried we were about him, how he was the center of our universe at that time and how much we loved him. Then I realized – what was more important is how his mind and his body must have been adapting and struggling for survival – learning to survive in the world outside of the womb.

It was only his second day of life and he had a long battle in front of him that we did not know too much about at that time. I sat in the rocking chair and watched in the silence that was occasionally interrupted with the beeping of monitors. It was so silent that I could almost hear myself breathe. My restless mind kept going and I just wanted it to stop worrying for a while.

I tried the ancient technique of taking three deep breaths in a row and sat absolutely motionless for a while. I was so tired, I wanted to sleep but the last few times I tried to sleep, I couldn't! The restless mind kept me awake. I looked at Rajan sleeping and I wished I could just go into a world of sleep like this little baby without thinking of anything at all.

Just then a nearby monitor beeped and brought me back to my nervous, anxious and worried state of mind. Soon I was reminded by the nurse that it was time for shift change at the NICU and that all parents needed to leave the unit for half hour. In the course of the next month, this schedule registered in my mental calendar just like recess does in a school student. I walked out of the NICU with a blank mind.

"What should I do next?" I thought to myself. Is there a handbook that has guidelines on what next steps parents should be taking when they are in a situation like this? I felt the strong clasp of uncertainty on my mind. I stopped by Sheri's room and she was sleeping – her body craving the much needed rest. I wondered if her mind was actually resting. I decided not to go into the room. Instead I headed for the exit. I felt this temporary rush of adrenalin in me – driven by the curiosity to find out more about Rajan's condition and just try to figure out how exactly we could participate in this battle for survival and cure.

I drove the familiar roads to our house in an auto-pilot mode with my mind racing at a million thoughts a minute. I rushed home and went straight to the basement. To search / surf on the internet had become a basic trait in the lifestyle of the modern human being. It could very well be clubbed with other basic traits like the need to sleep, eat, think, etc. I typed the keywords and every keystroke felt like a dagger in my heart. Most Google searches yielded in results that were links to research articles written by physicians or surgeons.

I was specifically interested in the surgeons' articles, given the upcoming next step was surgery. I printed some more stuff to take with me to read. I also printed information describing the basic organs and functions of the digestive system. Through my academic exposure to the science of engineering and in my professional career as an engineer, I had learned to systematically establish a sense of a predictable order and structure in assimilation of relevant information and the prediction of a certain result with a given degree of reliability. Moreover, I had specialized in the science of quality engineering where using data, I had created a world of structure within chaos and unusual (special cause) events or results could be distinguished from the normal yet variable common cause situations.

I always thought about things in terms of processes and products. Products are usually the outcome of processes. However processes are viewed as a collection of events which may or may not be cyclic. In fact, a series of events are classified as a process typically if they are repeated at a given frequency.

The frequency aspect of the distinction is what makes it difficult to determine whether the sequence of events you are experiencing is unique or similar to other events that have happened with or without our (mankind) knowledge / acknowledgement of it. Yet, all this knowledge and experience felt irrelevant and useless at the time to me, as I was thrust into the world of medical care, and its processes and outcomes. I surmised that reading such papers may start helping me establish some sense of order and structure to the events that were happening around me.

It was time to head back to the hospital. Mavshi had made some parathas (Indian bread) along with some veggies. I quickly gulped down about four or five of them. I had been eating very fast without much regard to what I was eating – especially when I was in the hospital at the cafeteria. The body's reaction to stress is not the same in all people. Some experience high blood pressure, others get ulcers. In my case, it was extreme discomfort in my stomach and later in my bowels. Within fifteen to twenty minutes of eating, I could feel my stomach churning ungodly amounts of acid. I could feel the acid burn all the way through to my throat. It seemed like no matter what I ate, my digestive imbalance had a way to make every ingestion of food turn into physical and mental distress.

I drove to the hospital, placed my reading material in Sheri's room and before it I knew it, it was time to return to the house because Roshan needed me by him as he was about to go to bed. I wondered if going back and forth for just getting Roshan to bed was justifiable or reasonable and quickly determined that there was no correct choice in matters like this. It is what you feel appropriate in that instance of time. I decided to brave the chilly winds in the parking lot to get to my car, drove home and went through the sequence of events that could now be classified as a process given its cyclic nature.

I laid in bed with him until he fell asleep while trying to not get myself too comfortable. I needed to get up and drive back to the hospital. I was a divided soul. Half my family was in the hospital and the other half at home. The same popular songs played on my preferred radio station as I drove into the parking lot of the hospital. Not too many cars were on the first floor – the floor with a direct entrance to the hospital passage way to the main building.

As much as I wanted to, I was physically and mentally unable to gather the strength to go to see my son on the third floor. I barely made it to Sheri's room that was now dark. Contrary to my expectations, she was actually awake. In her half dazed state she asked me the same question everyone had been asking me since Rajan was born, "How is our baby doing?" I told her that I had not seen him in the last few hours and that I was coming straight from home.

Sheri could sense the fatigue in my voice and I told her that I would go and see him first thing in the morning. Given that it was only me who could have gone to visit him then, I pushed myself to go to the NICU even if it was for a few minutes – let my sore eyes see him resting, and to tell him that we loved him before going back to the room to try to get some sleep. I did just that and returned to Sheri's room. Without attempting to change into the comfortable pajamas that I had brought in my previous trip to the hospital, I didn't bother changing, but rather laid down, pulled the sheets and blanket over me and fell right to sleep in that uncomfortable cold hard sleep chair.

Mama (Sheri) with Rajan

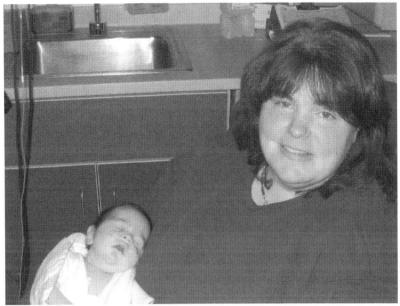

Baba (Devesh) with
Rajan

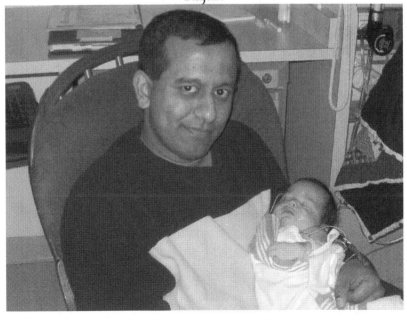

CHAPTER 7: SUNDAY – ANYTHING BUT A FUN DAY

It was Sunday afternoon. In our tired groggy states, our worry and frustration was building by the minute, partly attributed to lack of sleep and mostly to lack of information on what to expect (in the next few days and in the long term future). Out of the blue, there came a knock on the door followed very quickly by footsteps and right in front of us stood Dr. G. He greeted us, and in response to our surprised expressions of seeing him on a Sunday afternoon, began to talk about Rajan. We were told he was gone and not available for the weekend, but then again, it was getting close to the end of the weekend.

Apparently, Dr. G was back from whatever engagement he had and was doing his rounds and preparing himself for the upcoming work week. In a matter of fact tone, he mentioned logistics and schedule for the next day relative to Rajan. He told us that Rajan's surgery was scheduled for the early afternoon but had apparently gotten pushed to the last surgery of the day. I failed to understand how and why that decision was made.

Dr. G went on to explain that there were other more urgent cases (when severity and urgency are both high, the urgent cases almost always tend to win and take preference) that needed to be operated first. In a confident tone, he remarked that he was kept well informed by the team of Rajan's status, and would make any urgent changes to the planned schedule if his condition changed and required him to do so.

He concluded with the same "He is still stable and we continue to monitor him" statement that I was almost becoming allergic to, by this time. After he left the room, Sheri and I were left by ourselves in the quiet room that hummed lightly with the sound of the central HVAC. Sometimes, an apparent truth just seems to become more obvious and visible and here it was, the fact that our baby was born, but not with us, not in our room, not in our sight. In light of this feeling we had over the last two days, it just seemed to affect the core of our existence.

On day 2 of his life, his peripheral IV was replaced by a central venous catheter. *This is an IV port that is inserted through the arm and travels through a vein terminating in the inferior vena cava which is the gateway of de-oxygenated blood entering into the right ventricle of the heart – a high volume and high traffic blood junction in our body. If there is a spot that is guaranteed to take you places in your body, this is it.*

This is a routinely performed, nevertheless complex procedure, and we knew nothing about it. The way the hospital did this was that they asked for a quick permission, did the procedure and then informed us that it was completed. In our subsequent journey with children's hospitals, we found out through experience, that the children's hospitals are designed to deliver care to children with a lot more transparency, communication and involvement of the families rather than just administering the treatment to the patient with brief "FYI" communication to parents (which seemed to be the predominant style of this adult hospital).

CHAPTER 8: LONG OVERDUE

Another night passed and I woke up with a sore back when I realized that I had slept the night in a curled position on the sleeper-chair. It was a brand new day and a very crucial one. I kept looking at my watch and since nothing concrete had transpired yet, just kept re-assuring myself that it was still Monday. It was day three of his life and regardless of how you put it, Rajan's abdomen was essentially ballooning – a closed loop system with no outputs and toxic levels rising within the body by the hour. In the meanwhile, like clockwork, the notice for discharge on day three after child birth came through to us and this meant that Sheri would no longer have a hospital room to rest in. She was not critical, but was by no means in a position to handle this crisis.

The normal practice would have been to go home and rest / relax and enjoy our new baby. The latter part was not true, in fact we had no end in sight, just the realization that next big step was "Surgery". When the nurse brought Sheri's discharge papers to sign, I explained our situation and requested for the hospital room to be retained for Sheri for at least one more day, in order for her to have a place to rest.

The nurse remarked that she would be back after checking on the options. After a few minutes she returned with semi-optimistic news and stated that we had the room through the night, but not the next morning. We graciously accepted what we were offered, knowing that our energy and focus needed to be on Rajan, and his next steps of life. Our next question was regarding what time the surgery was scheduled and she replied immediately stating that we would receive that information from another source / department / personnel.

The hospital looked busy and nurses, doctors, patients and visitors swarmed in and out of the doors between the hallway and the maternity ward. Sheri came in and out of sleep induced by fatigue and pain medication drugs. I looked at my watch and it was just past noon, and we had not yet heard an update. I rang the bell and demanded that someone come and talk to us.

About an hour later (assuming most staff had gone to lunch), a resident showed up and gave us an update in the following words "A number of critical surgeries have come up and the two operating rooms are expected to be occupied for a significant amount of time, but we will do everything we can to get him scheduled. In the mean while… we are monitoring him and he seems to…" I interrupted him and protested stating that this was completely unacceptable and that I was not happy with what I heard and demanded to speak to the surgeon himself. The resident left the room without a troubled expression and I was not too concerned about whether I sounded courteous or polite given the gravity of the situation and the escalation of nerves we were experiencing.

Not much happened in the next couple of hours. Days and nights just seem to blur and merge into one another. There seemed to be only two things that occupied my entire day. I had a schedule of "in hospital" and "at home" time which was pretty much seamlessly transitioned from one to another with a heavier emphasis on the "in hospital" time and presence. I checked my watch and noticed that it was almost 4:30 pm. Before I could push the button to ask for assistance, the nurse showed up and gave me the list of medications Sheri would need.

They technically gave her discharge but allowed us to stay as late as we wanted through the night with availability of the room. The surgeon was supposed to come pay us a visit and brief us with an update on where things were. Frankly, we were not interested in an update but rather action involving getting him operated on – which by the book should have been done two days ago! Sheri and I then headed to the NICU to see Rajan.

While we were still waiting on the visit / update, I told Sheri that I was going to go to the pharmacy downstairs and get her medications, since the hospital pharmacy was about to close in half hour and I did not have the time to spare to go anywhere outside the hospital that evening. Going to the pharmacy downstairs for a few minutes was not a big deal in terms of making a decision, but as luck would have it, it actually was. The risk was that I could miss talking to the surgeon if, for whatever reason he showed up in exactly the time window for which I was away – the countermeasure for which was that Sheri was still in the room and available to talk. I stepped out of the room and rushed to the pharmacy downstairs hoping that Murphy's laws hopefully would not apply to this situation.

Down at the pharmacy, I handed over the prescription and my insurance information to the pharmacist. She was able to complete the prescription transaction fairly easily, but when it came to processing the insurance transaction, things became complicated. "What is it about medical insurance in this country that makes the incidence rates of confusion, rework, frustration and customer dissatisfaction seem to rate the highest amongst the various professions?" I thought to myself.

Isn't it ironical that the word "insurance almost inevitably brings negative thoughts to our mind when in reality the word should be responsible for creating a feeling or perception involving the concepts of "peace of mind", "coverage when you need it most", etc. However, now, of all times I hoped for the pharmacist and the insurance company to be my friends and not foe! She asked me a bunch of questions related to the insurance card and I answered mechanically looking for the end point of this process that results in medications in hand so I could rush back to where I was needed most. With the computer system not cooperating with the insurance information she was entering, she proceeded to then pick up the phone and try to talk to an insurance company representative.

I couldn't believe that I was going through all this for some standard medications after having used my existing active insurance card throughout the entire year on various occasions. After three to four long minutes of being on hold, she determined that she would somehow get the transaction processed. I demanded to get the medication so I could get out of there in the next minute or two regardless of whether insurance covered it or not. I wanted to tell her "My wife who wasn't doing so well is by herself upstairs in the NICU watching over our son; the surgeon operating on our son is supposed to show up any minute and my son's condition was in a constantly deteriorating state until surgical intervention was performed".

But instead I told her "Can you do whatever it takes and get me the medication NOW? I have to be upstairs to be briefed on a very important decision affecting my son's life. Within the next sixty seconds, I was handed some medication that included pain relief and antibiotics.

I signed the release form and ran with the medication in my hand to the elevator which was about to close. The elevator was occupied by a couple of middle-aged ladies that looked like nurses or technicians and a guy who looked like a maintenance worker. On the ride upstairs, all I could think of - was the hope that the surgeon had not showed up yet. Medications in hand, I walked with almost the pace of a decent jog to get to the room.

As I pushed the curtain aside, I saw Sheri in tears! All kinds of negative thoughts filled my already exhausted brain that was on the verge of explosion. "What's the matter?" I blurted in response to which she told me what had transpired in the last 20 minutes. As I listened to the events that had occurred, my fingers clenched and my fist shivered nervously. The surgeon had shown up exactly at the time that I was downstairs at the pharmacy. He had informed Sheri of a further delay in start time of the surgery and that he was going to go home and come back when the operating room was ready.

After hearing this, Sheri's brain had shut off to receive and comprehend any further information. As a response to this information, she had begun to cry uncontrollably and chose to neither acknowledge nor agree to understanding the course of action that the surgeon had just mentioned. Upon being asked if she had any questions or concerns (a rather rhetorical silly question to ask in a situation like this!) she had erred on the side of caution and mentioned that she was not in a position to reply and that it would need to be a joint response from her and me (when I returned).

I held Sheri's hand and managed to show an outwardly appearance of calm and reassured her "You did the right thing. I will speak to the nurse and ask if he is still here and hopefully we will be able to talk with the surgeon together before he leaves". In the back of my mind, the most recent sequence of events and communication seemed to be headed in the wrong direction.

Before I had a chance to get up, the surgeon re-entered the NICU. I wasn't sure whether to feel relieved and happy (that we got to talk to him before he left) or angry (couldn't he have waited to discuss this with the both of us instead of blurting out the news of the delay to the mother of a child who is struggling with coming to grips with dealing with the news of having delivered a child who has a birth defect?). But then again – in the busy life of a surgeon who is juggling several dynamically changing situations, anticipating the reaction of a mom (who happened to be by herself at that time) to news of delay in surgery of her new born son, was arguably not on the top of his priority list.

In the next few minutes, he described the helpless scenario of not being able to operate on Rajan because of the continued unavailability of the O.R because of being occupied on account of the unexpected arrival of two gun-shot victims at the hospital, who were being operated on an emergency basis. As I heard the words, the hypothetical scenarios of choice of human life and prioritization and logic seemed to have an eerie resemblance to my situation. The rational part of my brain did not seem to light up when a logical comparison was to be made.

My brief research on the internet on the subject by Dr. Alberto Peña from the previous day already had me thinking about how wrong all this was starting to seem to me, because the protocol had called for the operation of colostomy to be done shortly after 24 hours of birth for a case like this. From what I could remember, there was not much information in that article about the effects of not doing the surgery shortly after 24 hours, other than meconium build up. With my naivety about medical information (especially disorders), I had not known what meconium was nor had I the time to research it then either.

It was still not the age of widespread internet availability on phones and my searches were limited to the desktop computer at home. I gathered enough courage to say, "It's not that I don't care about the gun- shot victims, but what's happening with my son is NOT OK, and I want to know how soon my son can get into the OR and I am sick of waiting and sick of hearing "still stable" as justification for tolerating delays. I WANT ANSWERS NOW!"

The surgeon agreed and acknowledged the concern and echoed his frustration with the situation regarding availability. *(It would be many years and situations later, that I would learn about the increased emphasis of operations research in hospitals and its true value in terms of its impact on human beings).* He declared that he would be talking to the scheduling people and demanding an OR within a few hours and then he was gone.

I felt sick to my stomach about the helplessness I was experiencing. Was I under-reacting to the delays? What should I do? Should I yell? Cause a scene? Would that help or would it hurt and make the situation worse?

I felt my heart race as my body went into another episode of "fight or flight" type of response from the primal instinctive portion of my brain. I called Mavshi and provided my uncertain answer of the estimated time of surgery to her and checked on how Roshan was doing. How did we go from coming in for a known and scheduled C-section delivery for my wife to a required surgery for our new born child?

Saying the word "surgery" tugged hard on my emotional strings and seemed to try to weaken my will a little bit each time I heard it. I had not yet learned to fight... I felt like the weak unprepared scared 160 lb. amateur in a boxing ring with a seasoned mean 250 lb. muscled ruthless giant... and all I could think of was ... How did I get into this ring? I wanted to run... but there was nowhere to go... the lights shone brightly on us and my only real option was to fight... Back in Sheri's hospital room, a knock at the door and rustling of the curtain snapped me out of my daydream that seemed to be very reflective of my situation in real life.

As the white noise of the HVAC filled the room with a low but constant static, four hours had passed. It was only slightly brighter in the room compared to the outside where it was quite dark except for the diffused lights from the outside lighting of the hospital and the parking lots. They had come to inform us that it was time to take Rajan to the O.R.

Within minutes, Sheri and I were at the NICU and walked with our baby being carried to the OR on the oversized gurney. He looked so small and vulnerable and now distinctly bloated (which made me mad – because it certainly was because of the delay). For a moment, I thought about the mechanics of the situation. Although somewhat of a crude analogy, his body was essentially acting like a pressure vessel with an ever increasing buildup of internal pressure with no opportunity for relief.

I thought about how difficult it was for me to acknowledge and try to describe the nature of the defect to my parents and my brother and my sister in law. The social environment was already affecting my ability to deal with the situation. Why is it that a hole in the heart or a deformity in an appendage like toes or fingers is understood and perceived so differently, than an anomaly in genitalia or portions of the lower GI tract? There was much to learn about the social aspects and implications this would bring in the years to come that I had no idea about, at this time. This was just the beginning of the journey and the learning.

CHAPTER 9: THE COLOSTOMY

After what seemed to feel like eternity, we were suddenly at the point where it felt certain that Rajan was now scheduled and about to go into the Operating room. We were informed that the time of the surgery was going to be at 9:00 pm on Monday, almost 80 hours after he was born (well outside of the recommended post 24 to 30 hour guideline… this deviation from the guideline bothered me even while I did not fully comprehend the clinical aspects of it mostly because it seemed wrong). At 8:30 pm Sheri and I were with Rajan in the pre-operating waiting room waiting for the surgeon to arrive. Now every serious aspect of the situation started to sink into my conscious realization.

While I was furious about him not being operated on soon enough, now my mind craved more time… more time because the delay would seem comforting seemingly in an attempt to avoid the inevitable …and the inevitable event was the surgery. We had been briefed about this surgery earlier during the afternoon. When a child is born without the anal opening (imperforate anus), depending upon the severity of the situation, an intervention is required.

After reviewing the X ray revealing the anatomy of the rectum, Dr. G had concluded that Rajan was born with the congenital (at birth) defect of "high" imperforate anus. This meant that the position of the rectum was much higher in the body than where it needed to be. To correct this defect, there would be the need for an extensive surgery which was not recommended at this stage. Instead, a surgery providing a temporary solution and relief to the problem was going to be performed. This surgery was called "Colostomy".

It dealt with making an incision into the abdomen and cutting the distal portion of the colon and pulling it up and outside the body (skin) to provide it an opening for stool to exit the body. The brief literature about Colostomy provided pictures showing what to expect. However, our attention was so focused on Rajan and our minds so preoccupied with disbelief, that our comprehension of the material about the surgery was quite limited. I couldn't believe all this was happening. I just wanted this to be over for everything to return to normal as soon as possible.

At long last after an anxiously excruciating delay riddled with inexcusable reasons like unavailability of the surgeon and then the operating room, the surgery was finally under way. We sat in the waiting room. It was our first experience of waiting in the surgical waiting room of this hospital and also the first experience of awaiting the outcome of surgery for our child. In the life of the modern busy non-medical family, the closest thing to experiencing anything like this would be watching medical reality TV shows and other dramatized medical TV shows like Gray's anatomy.

Waiting is an interesting phenomenon. By definition it involves passage of time in anticipation of a (desired / expected) result. It also generally has an element of helplessness associated with it as it applies to the person / people waiting for the result. It may seem like it is only the patient and family who has to wait. But think about it... everyone seems to be waiting for varied periods of time before they can do anything meaningful or value added.

Even the seemingly precious resource in the form of the surgeon and his team experienced a significant amount of waiting time because the operating room was not available. However, there is also another distinguishing characteristic about the waiting time.

When patients and families wait in the waiting rooms before they are seen by the nurse and doctor in a clinic room setting, there seems to be a lot more "irritation" experienced than when compared with the waiting for the result of the surgical outcome. The primary difference comes from two factors – a) the gravity of the situation and b) in the latter case, you are waiting while important work is being done on **your** loved one. As we waited in the waiting room, I did what I could to comfort Sheri who at the time was not doing so well. What else might one expect from a mother coming straight from having surgery in the delivery room to waiting in the surgical waiting room to hear news about her new born baby? Clearly there was a vast departure from the norm and this was only the beginning of the unknown journey we were chosen to embark on.

These were not matters of choices or for that matter the consequences of choices made. In a vast majority of cases, these anomalies were random, unexplained and rude surprises to the parents of the newborn baby. *At that very moment, I had learned to NOT label such babies as "unfortunate". It was ok for the world to use the term – for instance, to use it in the context of a fund raiser for better care delivery or research for cure and treatment. But this word had no place in our acceptable vocabulary because it belonged in the camp of abettors of the enemy. The "enemy" was a vague illusion of a strong reality and its shape and form would emerge and manifest itself through the symptoms of the malformation and the associated disease it would bring. The loosely defined enemy always brings chills to my body because I know that the enemy is stealthy and evil by the nature of its being. The word "unfortunate" strongly supports the word helplessness and the feeling of helplessness was without a doubt in the enemy camp. I had to understand this better – this was the beginning of a war. The war would have several battles and some battles would be unannounced and others would have an expected outcome of "build up" of undesirable phenomena.*

The minutes turned to hours and the wait was over when the silence in the room was interrupted by footsteps and a rustle of scrubs. Dr. G had come to meet with us and give us news about the surgery. As he spoke, for some crazy reason, my eyes drifted to his fingers which appeared thicker / fatter than the norm. I wanted to focus very hard and the harder I tried, the more it was escaping me. I had formed an opinion of this doctor and it was interfering with my ability to listen to what he was saying.

Despite the mental barrier, we both listened intently as he gave us an update on the surgery and on our son's status. He told us that the surgery had gone well and he was able to do the colostomy with the two stomas emerging from the skin in the abdomen. It was only then that I decided to look up the brochure about the colostomy and subsequently additional information about colostomies. *So, here's a little information about colostomies. They are essentially bypass systems created in the colon. Their nomenclature mostly depends upon the location of where the bypass is created, the number of openings brought to the surface of the skin and the time period over which it is intended (temporary vs permanent) and are functionally linked with the anatomy of the diseased / malformed portion of the colon. The types of colostomies performed are:*

1. ***Ascending colostomy*** *(opening created in the ascending part of the colon leaving only small active portion of the colon) this colostomy is rarely done and an ileostomy is preferred over this option for situations requiring this type of stool diversion.*

2. ***Transverse colostomy*** *(opening created from the transverse portion of the colon)*

   a. ***Loop transverse colostomy*** *– Fig. 3 (two stomas located close to one another – one from the active portion of the colon for waste removal and the other from the inactive portion for mucous drainage)*

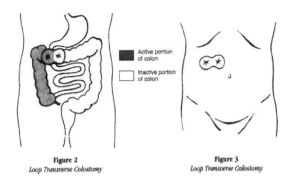

Figure 2
Loop Transverse Colostomy

Figure 3
Loop Transverse Colostomy

b. ***Double barrel transverse colostomy*** – *Fig 4 (a completely surgically divided colon usually resulting in two stomas similar to the loop colostomy; one from the active portion of the colon and the other from the inactive portion)*

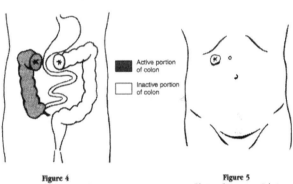

Figure 4
Double-Barrel Transverse Colostomy

Figure 5
Double-Barrel Transverse Colostomy

3. *Descending and sigmoid colostomy (made from the descending portion of the colon located in the lower-left quadrant of the abdomen, with separated stomas. The proximal stoma is connected to the upper gastrointestinal tract and drains stool. The distal stoma, also called a mucous fistula, is connected to the rectum and will drain small amounts of mucus material)*

Source: https://www.cancer.org/treatment/treatments-and-side-effects/treatment-types/surgery/ostomies/colostomy/types-of-colostomies.html

Dr. G had performed a descending/sigmoid colostomy with two visible stomas protruding on the left side of his abdomen. Sheri and I walked to the recovery room. Upon arriving at the recovery room, we realized that there is no amount of mental preparation or reading that could have ever truly prepared us to see the sight of our baby laying in a still manner which shook us to the core and struck the deepest chords of pain that we experienced for him.

From this point onward, we had embarked on a journey where we would be presented with several occasions where we would want to trade places with him and take away his pain and suffering. But we knew that we couldn't do that and the only thing we could do is love him intensely and offer all the care and support that we could possibly offer him.

Our baby was laying there, very still and connected to oxygen through a mask, to an IV in his arm and to cardiac and oxygen monitors through leads placed on his chest and toes. The wires and the equipment seemed to be overpowering, in comparison to his tiny body. Then we looked at his abdomen and noticed a bandaged and dressed area where the stomas were brought to the surface of the skin. There was also heavy bandaging across his abdomen in a transverse manner. It was a sight which takes a lot of courage to accept as reality. Indeed reality can be very cruel at times.

We sat by him gently touching his free arm (without the IV port). How would dealing with and recovering from a surgery work in conjunction with him growing as a new born baby (which by itself is such a complex, intricate, intense and aggressive phenomenon)? Would the developing network in his brain be able to handle all this extra stress of being under anesthesia, being operated on and having a portion of his colon bypassed?

While there was much for even experts to yet learn about the mysteries of human anatomy, pathophysiology of babies, I didn't want to ponder any more on this other than focus my attention on the basics of human life and caring. I could feel my primal instincts kick in as I thought and prayed intensely for survival, for the life of our baby. *Human babies are miracles of science and of humanity. They are so resilient on the one hand and also so delicate and fragile on the other. It is this mix and balance of the two extremes that makes everyone in the pediatric care delivery world fascinated about working in it.*

About a half hour later, Rajan was moved from the recovery room to the NICU. *A hospital stay for a loved one is kind of a unique phenomenon. The closest analogy is to that of a prison sentence or a rehabilitation center. There is hopefully (and in most cases) an expected end in sight. Many variables determine the length of stay. The cause for the hospitalization, the way the patient reacts, the rate at which they recover and then, of course, a vast world of unpredictable quality of care and circumstantial factors. You mostly have the attitude of doing your term and the strongest motivating factor is "getting out of there" – with a good outcome and an accompanying low probability of returning.*

Little did I know that as a chronic disease patient, we would be frequently visiting hospitals a lot more often than we would have liked to. Rajan's first surgery (descending colostomy) was performed on day 3 of his life. As every minute and hour passed, the clouds of uncertainty were kept at bay over the next day and on day 5, a remarkable event occurred.

His breathing had stabilized and they took him off his ventilator. But there always was this impending "fear" that reminded us of the fact that most hospital stays tend to be comprised of ups and downs as opposed to smooth sailing – a bit like being at sea on a cruise ship for a whole week. There will be at least one rough day at sea.

On day 9, more progress (seemingly) – antibiotics were discontinued. They also attempted oral feedings, but he did not seem to keep any feedings down. Later that night, he developed a fever – not a good sign, definitely not a good sign a few days post-surgery. He was given Tylenol for fever and a blood sample was whisked away to determine the source of the potential infection.

Infections are like ghosts (if you believe in them or appreciate the concept). You don't really see them but you see the effects of their actions in a very distinct way. They have a way of making their presence seen and felt through the person they affect.

CHAPTER 10: THE COMPLICATION

The fever did not subside, nor did our continuing apprehension and nervousness about the situation. The surgery had taken place and we had barely learned about the management of a colostomy and here we were… at a juncture of more impending danger. Unlike our previous episodes of conscious waiting, we were surprised by the surgeon's unexpected visit while we were at Rajan's bedside.

It was a Sunday afternoon and he was doing some unscheduled rounds to catch up with his patients before yet another most likely busy, hectic and unpredictable upcoming week. Dressed in his dark blue pants, crisp white shirt and signature "kids" tie, he evaluated Rajan's condition using the senses by touching the area near his still tender incision and specially the stomas.

Visually, things just did not look right. To add to the visual symptoms, Rajan also had a fever for the last day, and along with an unusual weight gain and an unexplained abdominal distension, there was also an irregular pattern of discharge from the mucous fistula. The skin near the distal stoma (mucous fistula - connected to the inactive portion of the colon) looked inflamed and the fistula looked half way recessed.

Dr. G ordered for a sample of the mucous fistula discharge to be sent for culture. We had barely recovered from the mental and physical exhaustion associated with our new reality. Then the news we dreaded came from the doctor. "One of the complications that can happen with this type of surgery is prolapse of the stoma created. Out of the two stomas, the mucous fistula has started to recess and I would like to re-operate as soon as possible" explained Dr. G.

He went on to provide statistics associated with the occurrence of the mucous fistula prolapse. At this point of time, we were least receptive to statistics since it was quite apparent that we were falling in the bucket of the unfavorable statistic lately for just about everything. Besides, would a higher or lower incidence of the occurrence of the complication make us feel better or worse?

Not really – it may make the surgeon feel better or worse, but is not likely to make the patient feel any different from the inevitable effect of the negative connotation of the complication. Dr. G went on to say that he would need to do another operation. With our scant understanding of this condition and its management, we were in no position to evaluate the connection of the complication with surgical skill, the propensity for complications, other care delivery aspects or uncontrollable biological aspects.

So we went with the flow, yet again succumbing to the pressure of the "what other options do we have or should consider?" feeling. Whatever crisis we were in, was far from over. The news of the need for another surgery was like telling a marathon runner to run another 10 miles after he finishes the marathon...or rather thinks he finished the marathon! I thought some more about the marathon analogy and although I did not know the true extent of the care that Rajan would require, I knew that we, as his parents and as care givers, would need to condition ourselves more like marathon runners rather than sprinters. Unlike the previous fiasco associated with the start time of the first surgery, the second surgery was planned and executed per schedule

Rajan's second surgery (a result of a complication developed from the first surgery) went smoothly, although of course we were still coming to terms with the word "complication". In reality, we were slowly but surely getting introduced to an imperfect and rather immature field of medical science and medical care delivery. It was a late Monday night as we waited yet again in the surgical waiting area. This time, we were the only people there as it was a rather late in the night.

For some reason, my brain related the waiting situation with waiting at a Greyhound bus station on a weekday night at a remote Midwest city. Perhaps, I was starting to just not expect good results and unconsciously making a biased judgment of the quality of care he was receiving. This conclusion did not have much of a rational basis at the time, since I had inadequate knowledge of good medical care delivery standards, and a relatively unknown idea of Rajan's realistic prognosis.

Approximately two hours after we saw Rajan being wheeled into the operating room, we now had some news. It was Dr. G, walking toward us, still in his scrubs, but with his cap and mask off. As our anxious hearts beat at least 20 beats per minute faster than normal, I tried to clear my mind to listen to what he had to say. "The operation went well", began Dr. G "and I was able to restore the stoma to the appropriate protrusion", he continued to explain to us. Our medically naïve brains at the time were functioning to simply extract key words and evaluating their implications on the optimism scale that arbitrarily went from a bad" to "good" continuum.

After the conversation, the conclusion in our minds was definitely past the midpoint on the continuum scale and leaning toward the "good side". We could expect the pointer to shift more, only after a visual confirmation upon actually seeing Rajan. We thanked the surgeon – a sincere thanks from my part, but with a large burden of "the unknown" that seemed to be choking me from the inside. We proceeded to go and see Rajan in the recovery room.

The sight of peripheral IV lines, leads connected to monitors and various other medical paraphernalia somehow fades into the distant background when it comes to the singular focus the brain hones in on, when it comes to assessing your child from a parent perspective. We first yearned to "feel" through our senses how he was doing. He lay there motionless, except for the steady and rhythmic expansion and contraction of his bare chest. For several minutes, I just watched him... letting my mirror neurons go into hyper-drive as I imagined how he must feel, while energizing the empathy circuits of my brain like never before.

While being connected to the mask that delivered oxygen, I felt in a strange way that his breaths and ours as parents were synchronized and that as long as we had breath and a beating heart, so would he and that nothing could ever get in the way of a successful recovery for him. As I was living in this "quasi-state" of mind, one of the monitors went off. I learned very quickly that monitors in the medical field were very similar to the various sensors that I was used to working with in the manufacturing engineering field.

We had sensors at just about every station on every manufacturing line. Just like how the science of measurement of health status through monitors was rather weak and neglected, so was the situation of sensors in core processing and testing machines on the assembly line. The sensors on the assembly line existed for one primary reason – to check, verify and report out on the status of something important. This usually translated to a key physical or functional characteristic of the product or a component of the product that was being manufactured.

As one of the nurses attended to the pulse ox sensor that had triggered the alarm, she first checked on the status of the lead connected to his toe and realized that it was not making good enough contact – which she attributed to the lower level of oxygen that had triggered the alarm on the monitor.

CHAPTER 11: THE DIARY OF THE FIRST MONTH

Consider the following medical experiment. The next couple of pages highlight a chronological diary of events and associated specifics across the timer period of Rajan's first month of life. The following few chapters, on the other hand are a detailed description of same on the form of a story. See for yourselves how your emotions and reactions vary as you see the unfolding of the story articulated in two different ways.

First month Diary of Rajan:

1. 12-03-04
    a. Born at 14:27 hrs at hospital (in Flint MI)
    b. Wt. 8 lbs 11 oz
    c. Length: 19.75 in
    d. Diagnosed with imperforate anus. Initial diagnosis by Dr.G. Conversation with the surgeon on the same evening.
    e. Blood tests, X rays and ultrasounds completed on same day
    f. Placed on IV same day
2. 12-04-04
    a. Central venous catheter placed in replacement of peripheral IV
    b. 12-06-04
    c. Colostomy surgery performed by Dr. G. at 23:45 hrs
    d. Duration of surgery : 25 minutes

    e. Dr. G concludes high imperforate anus condition

    f. Colostomy stoma and mucous fistula brought to the abdomen surface

    g. Started antibiotics

3. 12-08-04

    a. Ventilator removed

4. 12-11-04

    a. Oral feedings attempted – Not successful

    b. Antibiotics discontinued

    c. Developed high temperature (103) at night

    d. Antibiotics resumed

    e. Tylenol given for fever

    f. Feedings discontinued

    g. Blood sample given for culture to determine source of potential infection

5. 12-12-04

    a. Dr. G. examines baby

    b. Unusually high weight gain; significant abdominal distention; incision site shows signs of infection; Mucous fistula is recessed (prolapse); drainage of mucous is irregular

    c. One large discharge observed from mucous fistula – sample from discharge sent to culture to determine source of potential infection

    d. Dr. G. makes decision to re-operate to pull mucous fistula back to the surface

6. 12-13-04
   a. Second surgery (mucous fistula prolapse repair) performed by Dr. G. at 19:05 hrs
   b. Duration of surgery: 30 minutes
   c. Urinary bladder was enlarged and high in position due to excess urine retention
   d. Catheter inserted into urinary bladder for urine discharge
   e. Catheter added to mucous fistula to facilitate mucous discharge
   f. Bags attached to each catheter to monitor discharge from each

7. 12-15-04
   a. Ventilator removed

8. 12-16-04
   a. Oral feedings restarted; 5 cc Pedialyte doses

9. 12-17-04
   a. Two antibiotics discontinued — Ampicillin and Flagyl
   b. Meropenum to continue for another 7 to 10 days for fighting infection

c. Breast milk feedings introduced – starting at 5 cc with increments of 5 cc every two feedings Feeding frequency: 3 hours

d. Larger size catheter placed in mucous fistula

e. Urine leakage around urinary catheter is deemed OK according to doctor

10.   12-18-04

a. Feedings changed to 3 cc increments per feeding

b. Feedings are tolerated well in general

11.   12-21-04

a. Last antibiotic discontinued

b. I.V removed

c. Urinary catheter removed

d. Reglan medication started to reduce reflux

12.   12-23-04

a. Catheter in mucous fistula removed

13.   12-24-04

a. Continuous feed (25 cc per hour) started due to excessive vomiting and inadequate weight gain through NG tube

b. Reason: To determine cause of vomiting: whether it is the contents of the milk OR the ability to hold and digest large amounts of batched deliveries of milk

c. 3 weeks old today!

14.   12-27-04

a. Small oral feeds (25 ml every 4 hours) reintroduced

15.   12-28-04

a. Central venous catheter (I.V line) removed

b. Reglan dosage increased

c. Zantac dose stays the same

d. Oral feedings increased to 100 cc every 4 hours

16.   12-31-04

a. Water soluble liquid test with X ray performed

b. Dr. G. says distal end of colon is about 4 cm above bottom and corrective surgery is 8 to 12 months away

17.   01-01-05

a. Tongue tied condition detected by nurse and confirmed by doctor

b. Call put in for Dr. M. (ENT)

18.   01-02-05

a. Develops high temperature up to 103.5 F

b. Treated with Tylenol for fever

c. Blood drawn at 14:00 hrs for culture

d. Blood sample for CBC showed high WBC count (24)

19.   01-03-05

a. Dr. G. examines baby; suspects UTI (urinary tract infection); orders urine culture

b. Urine sample sent for culture

c. Referred to Dr. R. who starts him on antibiotics (gentamicin 16 mg every 24 hours and ampicillin : 400 mg every 8 hours) by I.V

d. Dr. M. repairs tongue tied condition

20.   01-04-05

a. Blood culture negative

b. Urine culture positive for bacterial infection (E-Coli)

21.   01-06-05

a. All agree; Rajan gets discharge and comes home!

b. Urine culture sent to lab

22.   01-25-05

a. Readmitted due to fever

b. Suspected UTI – confirmed upon admission

23.   01-28-05

a. Discharged from hospital with slight temperature

b. New antibiotic to be started the next day

24.   01-29-05

a. New antibiotic – Augmentin started

b. Very loose stool observed after a few days

25.   01-31-05

a. Appointment with Dr. A. (Pediatric infectious disease specialist)

b. Antibiotic changed to Ceftin

c. Did not do well with Ceftin — lots of vomiting

26.   02-02-05

a. Appointment with Dr. G. ; Dr. A. also present

b. Changed antibiotic to Suprax

c. Did well with Suprax

CHAPTER 12: TROUBLE DOUBLED

It was exactly 12 days since Rajan was born, and things didn't exactly seem to be settling down at all. That evening, upon one look at Sheri, I knew that she was not feeling well. As a matter of fact, she was getting very sick...by the minute. She and I knew that almost instantly and intuitively, even though we did not know what specifically was wrong. Her color looked pale, her energy level was low and she just wanted to sit on the rocking chair with her arms crossed while being covered under her favorite University of Michigan blanket. I called her OB/GYN doctor and described the symptoms. There was no hesitation from the doctor.

The doctor advised to get Sheri admitted ASAP. In less than half hour, we were in the emergency room at hospital H and a battery of tests began. It was a unique memory associated with the situation. The resident who was examining her, sparked a conversation about careers. As soon as I mentioned that I was an engineer, he commented that he was an engineer too. He went on to describe his journey of working in a company as an aeronautical engineer and then about his decision to change his career and go back to medical school.

I thought about the key characteristics that might be required for such a radical change:

a) *A strong desire to accomplish the objective / ambition*
b) *The will / courage to act upon that desire and have the persistence to pursue it*
c) *Circumstances (the mix of the favorable and opposing conditions) relative to the environment and its influence / effect on a) and b).*
d) *Destiny (the subset of circumstances that are extreme unexpected chance events which may have a profound positive or negative impact on the desire and the will.*

As I finished my train of "factors of influence" thought process, worry rose to astronomical levels in my head with the sudden realization that my wife and my son were in the hospital at the same time, and that situation just seemed too difficult to accept or swallow. One in the ER and the other in the NICU. This was by far one of the most challenging moments of my life.

I don't exactly remember how I was splitting my time or attention between taking care of my wife and my son in the hospital at the same time. With Rajan being somewhat stable and knowing that he was likely to be in the hospital for a long time, I knew that I had to focus on Sheri getting better, for her sake, for my sake and for our sake so we could together focus on getting Rajan out of the hospital and on the road to a "normal / healthy" life, although of course we were still trying to figure out what that would look like or mean for him. While my mind was grappling with the stress associated with the uncertainties of Rajan's tumultuous experience in the hospital, I could really not fathom how I was going to be able to handle and manage the complexities of care that were likely to emerge from Sheri's hospitalization.

For the first time, I felt terrified by thoughts of losing my family. It is times like these that the physical presence of family or friends in that moment and situation can be so helpful. Although I had support from Mavshi who was at home with Roshan and my parents and my brother and his family (who were still physically continents away), I felt very alone in that situation challenged with two of my family members in the hospital at the same time.

A few hours into the hospitalization, the doctors were conducting a flurry of tests and the cause of biggest concern was the condition of her heart. She had been on steroids for management of her acute asthma attacks. But now, they were suspecting some form of heart enlargement as a part of postpartum stress. She was also retaining a lot of fluid resulting in high blood pressures. She was under close observation, but getting the edema under control seemed to be the logical first step which they began working on – right away. This in turn was expected to have cascading changes that would bring about the much needed homeostasis*.

As the diuretics and other meds worked in combination, she began to get some relief and so did I. As the number of stressors increased, my own body reacted and did so primarily in the form of severe stomach upsets and heartburn. Often I would wake up with heartburn and it would lead me to believe that food choice had nothing to do with how I was feeling. As I battled my nervous stomach, I had to keep my focus and hope on Sheri feeling better. Appropriate care, her own determination and my love and prayers got her to the point where the hospital was ready to let her go home.

A huge sigh of relief and happiness surged through my entire body. As I looked at her though, something still didn't seem right. There was a form of unhappiness / distress that seem to engulf her entire being. She and I both knew that this was attributed partly to the obvious cause of being worried about our son, but also partly because of her postpartum hormonal imbalance. In our next visit to the ob-gyn, we didn't need to bring up the topic. The doctor herself did.

She first apologized and confided that she should have raised this topic and concern proactively – especially in light of the situation we were in. Recovering after a C-section delivery while your baby is still in the hospital and undergoing lifesaving surgeries seemed like an unsurmountable challenge. The ob-gyn realized that it certainly was a missed opportunity on her part to have anticipated a breakdown of the recovery process for Sheri.

A little more frequent monitoring may have saved us an emergency visit. Also, she asked the inevitable question of how Sheri felt (mentally) and brought up the topic of depression. We both agreed that we were at the point where, Sheri could benefit from being on a low dose of anti-depressant as we got through this situation. This was the first ever instance of being on such a medication and while we had our concerns about being on this medication, we allowed the potential short term benefits outweigh the potential risks and were very clear about having a near-term end date of the medication.

CHAPTER 13: THE NEW NORMAL

Days went by and for a little while, Rajan being in the hospital started to feel like the norm. This could very well be affected largely by the fact that he had not yet left the hospital since he was born. Many days, it felt as though he would never get out of the hospital.

During the first three weeks, his intake was not so good. So, an NG tube was placed through which we would feed him. While, entry into his stomach was easy, bypassing the mouth and esophagus creates unique and interesting challenges to the body of a baby and we got to see them first hand. The rate at which we entered the feeds and the amounts we entered mattered a lot. Also, bypassing salivary amylases* added challenges with retaining and digesting.

The biggest challenge to overcome was the timing of the break between feeds. We learned just the right position to hold him and try to burp him so that he kept the food down. It is amazing to see how the human bond makes its presence felt and realized through physical contact no matter how many leads or tubes may be connected to your baby. As related human beings, we always clung to each other. We hoped that the protective arms of mom and dad made all worries melt away even if it was for fleeting moments during his challenging journey.

Feeding and nutritional progress continued to be measured through daily weight recordings and through slow increases in oral feeds accompanied by slow decreases in tube feeds. All this seems obvious and logical; but every setback in the progress seemed so hard to swallow.

Immediately following surgery, abdominal distention was observed and then immediately acted upon by placement of a urinary catheter. Much of what I was observing felt like watching a "Truth or fiction" show. Being at my lowest levels of medical literacy- oversights, mistakes and negligence mixed in with appropriate care was so indiscernible that helplessness seemed to be making a more prominent place in the emotional center of my brain and joining forces with despair and anxious uncertainty.

The neurological hormonal cocktails were having a field day as every day felt like a mine field of obstacles to tackle just to "stay alive". A catheter was also inserted into the mucous fistula. The urinary catheter and the catheter inserted into the mucous fistula were both individually and separately bagged to monitor urinary and mucous discharge respectively. The month of December seems to have its own unique pace – a pace different from other months – mostly attributed to its build up toward the last week of the month which also coincides with the last week of the year.

The hospital accelerated with its own build-up of decorations and festive fervor as the days of December passed by. Exactly in the middle of the month, a big milestone came about – his ventilator was disconnected since it was no longer required – a very positive sign in the direction of recovery and the prospect of discharge from the hospital. The following day, oral feeding resumed with a modest 5 ml pedialyte doses.

Yet another cloudy December day passed and marked the discontinuation of two antibiotics- Ampicillin and Flagyl. For precaution, it was determined to keep the ultra-broad spectrum Meropenem to guard against infections for another 7 to 10 days.

Little did we know that the word "infection" was going to be haunting us for almost a decade to follow. Then for the first time, we introduced breast milk feedings in very small quantities starting with 5cc and increments of 5 cc with each feeding that was executed with the precision of hospital frequency of every 3 hours.

The normal healthy baby goes through the simple cycle of eat, sleep and poop. But here we were – making our little introduction of breast milk to a child who had seen more anesthesia, antibiotics, diagnostic tests, catheters, leads and IVs in the first two weeks of his life than most people would encounter in their entire lifetimes.

CHAPTER 14: SMALL GLIMMERS OF HOPE

One thing was clear- each day was calibrated with changes – many in the direction of recovery and few that were set backs. However, it was the week of an unmistakable feeling of "net positive" changes! You didn't need to count them, the automatic mental math was reflecting itself in the small but highly treasured emphatic dopamine releases that made every single day feel better than the previous.

Growth – the often miraculous phenomenon that is taken for granted too often, made its presence felt when we moved a size up on the catheter that drained from mucous fistula. Every sign of growth and every discontinuation of a medicine began a metamorphosis of the mental mix of emotions. On the 18th day of December the feeding regimen was changed to incorporate 3 cc increments per feed and the "so far so good" feeling was experienced in the long breaths of relief that we enjoyed as we exhaled the hospital air. The next four days brought about the following four changes

a. Last antibiotic discontinued

b. I.V line removed

c. Urinary catheter removed

d. Catheter from mucous fistula removed

e. Reglan medication started to reduce reflux

While we continued our streak of net positive changes, the last change was a caution flag. We had to reintroduce continuous feeds (25 cc per hour) through the NG tube due to excessive vomiting and inadequate weight gain. The objective was to determine whether it was the contents of the milk or the ability to hold and digest large amounts of batched deliveries of milk that were causing the vomiting and hence inadequate weight gain.

The "net positive" changes in the past week had also led us to start believing that "Christmas" celebration at home with the whole family, was starting to become a possibility. However, Christmas Eve had arrived and while we had to give up on the hope of a discharge before Christmas, we also celebrated our little one's milestone of having turned 3 weeks old. As we reflected back on the three weeks, it felt the equivalent of three decades of struggle and every little victory along the way made the burden of anxiety and uncertainty a little more bearable as we looked forward to the light at the end of the tunnel.

Christmas came and went like just another day and no amount of decoration in the hallway leading to the NICU seemed to come even close to the sadness and emptiness that was filling my heart. The simple pleasures of being together as a family, hiding presents and then opening them in the morning, and enjoying Christmas dinner together as a family – all those things that I felt I had only semi-enjoyed in the past because of the element of just taking them for granted, now haunted me.

The family was fragmented, half at home and half in the hospital and for the first time, family togetherness gained a level of importance and appreciation that I had never experienced before. The undeniable power of circumstances had made it clear that the family was going to go through this stressful separation in an almost "God's will" sort of way.

So I accepted it and worked through it and rejoiced at the fact that there were still a few things that were in my control. It was a family tradition to buy an new ornament each year for the tree and was also a family tradition to make the ornament personally customized if we were to have any forms of additions to the family during the time of the holidays – for example family / guest visiting or like in this case a new bundle of joy entering our lives.

Despite the crazy schedule, Mavshi, Roshan and I had made it to the famous "world's largest Christmas store-Brunner's" which was only about 40 minutes' drive and had purchased a customized bulb with the words "Rajan" painted on it. I continued shuttling Sheri back and forth from home to the hospital and occasionally other family members made it with me on the trips to the hospital. While Christmas just didn't feel like a regular joyous Christmas this year, we did take a few minutes to sit and relax in the living room by the tree before it was time to head back to the hospital that day.

If there is such a thing as the feeling of being "torn", then I couldn't think of something more powerful than what I was feeling at that moment in time.

CHAPTER 15: IMPROVEMENT MOMENTUM

Two days later, the positive reinforcement cycle changes made their presence felt like the rays of light full of hope making their way between the dark clouds of despair.

a. *Small oral feeds (25 ml every 4 hours) reintroduced*

b. *Central venous catheter (I.V line) removed*

c. *Reglan dosage increased*

d. *Zantac dose maintained as same*

e. *Oral feedings increased to 100 cc every 4 hours two days later...*

The December build up to the end of the year had continued on and there it was -New Year's eve! While so much had changed and was continuing to evolve, there was the feeling of "not much has changed – SIGNIFICANTLY", since we had not realized and enjoyed the feeling of being home together as a family. On the last day of December a few important events occurred:

1. A water soluble liquid test with X ray was performed using the mucous fistula (this is my best description of the test as of my knowledge in the year 2004. Now I know so much more about water soluble distal colostograms and its significance in determining the success of a following PSARP – thanks to the detailed explanations written by Dr. Peña and Dr. Bischoff that were published 12 years later in 2016)

2. Based upon the test results, Dr. G announced that the distal end of colon is about 4 cm above his bottom and corrective surgery will be conducted in the next 8 to 12 months.

Along with this news, I also made the following resolutions:

In my mind, I announced to myself – "Starting today, I will change something about me – the helplessness and the deep anxiety resulting in deep despair gut wrenching disappointment will be eliminated and replaced with the following:

a. Never give up – even in the seemingly most hopeless sounding situations, there is a way to find a solution and to believe in it even if it may not be available and obvious at that time

b. Learn any and everything there is to know about a condition, if you want to overcome it. There was no way that I was going to let my non clinical academic background come in the way of my learning of the anatomic, physiologic and psychologic aspects of this condition that could help me in any possible way to make our son's outcome better.

c. Challenge everything and insist on learning "why" something was being done or not. Actions and inactions (in association with the timing of their execution or lack thereof) would become the foundation of a **joint** understanding of us and the medical team when it came to any medical decisions that would affect the life of our child in the future.

Then the New Year (2005) arrived. I was trying not to think too much about the fact that New Year's Eve was also experienced in a non-typical way with the hospital being a central part of the experience. I believe it was a fact that it was probably the most important part of our lives and it needed all the attention it deserved.

A couple of days before the end of the year, we were also informed of an observation that was related to some abnormality in speech production and could have also been related to his compromised ability to create a sucking action (to drink). It was the condition of being "tongue-tied". Here is some basic information about this fairly common and easily treatable condition. In case of Rajan's situation, the symptoms seemed to make a lot of sense especially relative to the difficulties with sucking and swallowing related to his oral feeds.

Tongue-tie (ankyloglossia) is a condition present at birth that restricts the tongue's range of motion. With tongue-tie, an unusually short, thick or tight band of tissue (lingual frenulum) tethers the bottom of the tongue's tip to the floor of the mouth. A person who has tongue-tie might have difficulty sticking out his or her tongue. Tongue-tie can also affect the way a child eats, speaks and swallows, as well as interfere with breast-feeding.

A call was put in for the ENT surgeon to perform a simple procedure to fix this problem. The ENT surgeon was Dr. M and happened to be the husband of Sheri's OB GYN...indeed a small world. As we were starting to somewhat enjoy the "net positive" trends and changes, the second day of the new year came with a nasty surprise.

He suddenly developed high fever (spiking at 103.5 F). He was given Tylenol to keep the fever in check and we knew instinctively, something worse was going to follow. A blood draw took place at 14:00 hrs that day and the CBC showed high WBC count of 24. This telltale sign of infection now needed to be investigated for the source.

The next day, Dr. G examined Rajan and suspected a UTI (urinary tract infection) and ordered for a urine sample to be sent for culture. He also referred him to Dr. R (an infectious disease specialist) who immediately put him on antibiotics - Gentamycin 16 mg every 24 hours and Ampicillin (400 mg every 8 hours) by I.V – had to be placed back on this little baby who had just barely started to experience some relief from lines and meds.

We had almost forgotten about the tongue tied condition that we were told about a few days ago. On the third day of January, the ENT surgeon (Dr. M) came to his bedside and conducted a very simple procedure to essentially free up the range of motion of the tongue by making a very small incision. He brought with him a dispensable cautery tool which he used and within a couple of seconds, it was done. The tool helped with instant wound recovery and healing. We were able to watch this in action and it was fascinating to see the tool "glow" when it was used. It was small and in the shape and size of a thick pen or a small flashlight.

When the surgeon was done with the surgery, he had no use for the tool and about to discard it, when I asked if we could keep the tool- well, because it was cool and it was probably the only surgical tool that could potentially be saved as a memory or souvenir. The surgeon thought for a little bit and announced "Sure, as long as you promise to keep it away from children and be responsible with it and not use it on anyone. Although its power is reduced after its first use, it can still cause damage". We agreed and I quickly put it away into my backpack and we pretended as if this conversation and handing over of a tool that was supposed to be disposed of – did not happen at all.

Amongst what seemed like grim situations to deal with, I enjoyed this brief moment and winked as I looked at my wife with a sly smile. It was also the day that we had a little celebration – it was the 3rd. of January and Rajan had turned a month old. The nurse had created a little poster that stated "Rajan: Congratulations! Happy One Month Birthday!"

A nurse holding Rajan at Hospital H

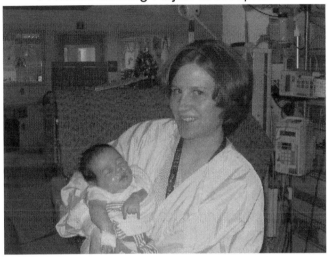

Rajan turns one month old, and has yet to leave the hospital since his birth.

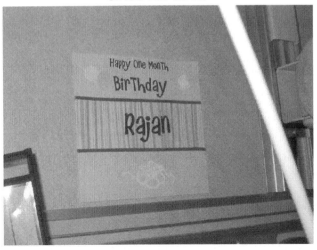

CHAPTER 16: HOMECOMING

The much awaited test results came in the following day. Blood culture negative (Whew!) and urine culture positive (as suspected) for bacterial infection (E-coli). This was my first exposure (from an awareness / knowledge standpoint) about infections...especially UTIs. Up to this point in my naïve mind, UTI was the infection that typically happened in women. But, now all common knowledge had to be set aside as we grappled with the reality of the term "anorectal malformation" and its effects.

So, for all practical purposes, we were in completely unchartered territory relative to our understanding of the disease and its treatments. *Speaking of general statistics, 85% of all UTIs are caused due to E-Coli bacteria (the generally harmless bacteria living in the gut that causes havoc when it finds itself in a different environment – like the urinary tract). Also, women are four times more likely to get a UTI than men – due to the anatomical differences directly related to the probability of entry of the gut bacteria into the urinary tract.* So – how did Rajan end up getting a UTI? I had no idea or understanding of the causes of this. But, I wanted to know "Why?" While all this was going on, tensions were rising.

An important question to answer was "Did he still need to be in the hospital?" It wasn't the first time, we approached this topic and question. But this time, Sheri was insistent. She had approached the doctor and asked for what it would take for Rajan to be released from the hospital.

The discovery of the most recent infection had not yet sunk in to our minds. We were not convinced about the connection of the treatment of infection with his need to be in the hospital. At this point of time, the overwhelming ambition and desire for all of us was to get out of the hospital. Sheri literally begged the doctor and asked what it would take. Over the past few weeks, we had already mastered the skills of colostomy care which included:

- preparing the stoma bag (cutting the appropriate size hole in the adhesive base of the bag)
- cleaning the area around the stoma
- placing the bag around the stoma to create a tight seal
- Watching out for inflation of the bag (as it collected stool and /or gas)
- Deflating it periodically (yes… this is the part where you would want to close your nose and hold your breath)
- Replacing the bag upon too much accumulation of stool or the indications of a leak

Also included in our training was demonstration of proper re-insertion of the NG tube and proper care of the other stoma (the mucous fistula). After a lot of convincing - primarily by Sheri and after several discussions of pro/s and cons, the doctor decided that it was ok for Rajan to be discharged. Despite all the difficulties we were facing, this decision by far was the first BIG victory for us all. It was time that Rajan stepped outside of the hospital, breathed the outside natural air – for the first time and most importantly come home and continue with his recovery. I distinctly remember the day when this decision was made (06-January 2005).

We had only one cell phone at the time that we shared between myself and Sheri. I remember Sheri calling me on the cell phone that morning from the hospital room phone as I was driving toward home and she exclaimed with joy "We get discharged today and we are going home!!!" I called Mavshi who was at home and we all couldn't contain our excitement about this fantastic news. It was a very strange and wonderful feeling I experienced. I rolled down the window and let the brisk January air blow in my face. It reminded me of the Jerry Maguire movie scene of when he quits his job and feels the excitement of starting a new journey as he blasts the song "Free falling…" on his car stereo. I looked outside the window and noticed a large bird doing a sort of dance in the air – not exactly flying but just floating and using the gusts of the wind and its wings to dive and soar and just "be" in the moment. For the first time, I learned what it was to just be and live in the moment…it was a moment like I had never experienced before. It was also a moment where I realized a very different kind of joy.

All my life thus far, I was used to the kind of joy that was almost exclusively linked with me or my accomplishments. But on this day, I experienced wonderful and true joy for someone else…someone so dear to me that the joy I experienced was vastly superior to the joy I knew about from my past. It must have been an experience which my mind actually learned and stored in a part of my brain such that I was able to feel it every subsequent time he was discharged from the hospital in the future years to come.

Instead of the normal 2 to 3 day stay in the hospital post-delivery, we were now going on 34 days post birth and here it was – the moment we had been waiting for – the day we would finally get to go home. On the one hand, it was great to breathe a sigh of relief to come home after successful completion of two surgeries including a life-saving one (for which we were grateful) and the feeling of having this whole month behind us. But on the other hand, the words "long and often bumpy road ahead" haunted and reminded me that the challenging journey that was far from over, had just begun!

CHAPTER 17: SETTLING IN

For the entire time that Rajan was in the hospital, I had been off work for the most part. I had attempted to go in for a few days, but it was too hard and on the days that I did end up going to work, extreme events relative to Rajan's and

Sheri's health deteriorations had forced me to abandon the idea and just pay attention to taking care of the family. I had also missed one day of the two day training class which was supposed to help me learn about the problem solving methodology that I was planning on using for my work project.

I was fortunate enough to have a great manager and colleagues at work who covered for me in my absence. Brief thoughts of losing my job crossed my mind, but I tried not to think too much of it. I had my priorities straight – the family in times of dire need always came first, but I didn't know how I would have thought about it if there were no concessions offered from work and if survival were to compete with providing care while taking time off.

When Sheri and I arrived home with Rajan for the first time, we were greeted by a nice "Welcome" sign made by Mavshi and Roshan. Mavshi wore the traditional sari that day to celebrate the auspicious nature and significance of the event. She had already made dinner and it was a special night as it was the first night that our newly expanded family was going to spend together at home.

In the weeks that followed, we provided all the necessary care that was required and his prescribed dose of antibiotic had exhausted. He seemed to tolerate oral feeds much better and the need for the NG tube was eliminated. His feeds involved a formula and breast milk mix to ensure that he was getting plenty of nourishment to sustain the required weight gain at this crucial stage of his growth as a baby.

After a long break, I resumed going back to work. During the next two weeks there were many appointments to keep, medications to be given, and fluid intake to be monitored. During the first week, a nurse visited our home three times, then twice during the second week – all part of the agreed upon protocol that we signed prior to discharge.

The hospitalization that Sheri herself had to undergo, and the subsequent recovery from it was difficult. She gave little importance to her own health as the focus was taking care of Rajan. This always made me nervous and I worried about her as much as I worried about Rajan. Sheri took him to these appointments by herself since I could not afford to take additional time off. Dealing with a C-section recovery followed by arrhythmia of the heart, post-partum depression, excessive fluid retention, the psychological trauma of taking care of a sick baby was taking a toll on her although she was not willing to admit it.

We had a follow up visit with the OB GYN and I accompanied her to the doctor visit. The doctor was aware of the situation with Rajan, but her main focus was now making sure that she was monitoring Sheri's condition closely. I would occasionally join them at the appointments if I could, by taking a couple of hours off during work. Rajan was doing better, but something just did not seem to feel right. There was not really a good explanation that the doctor had provided at the time for the UTI that had happened just before we had left the hospital. While we were treating it now, the feeling of unanswered questions was haunting me.

CHAPTER 18: READMISSION

Before we knew it, the 25th of January had arrived. Exactly three years ago, we had celebrated the arrival of our first son Roshan into this world. We had planned a small but nice "close family only" type of birthday celebration for him that year. But on this day, we had an early dinner and we planned to cut cake and have him open his presents in the evening. As Roshan was playing with the cool "Dinosaurs" that he had received as presents, Rajan became very fussy.

Rajan's color didn't look right. He felt warm to the touch. Upon checking with a thermometer, he was already at 101 deg. F, and it felt like things were about to get worse again. He had already received his last dose of scheduled antibiotic. We gave him some Tylenol and changed our metal status to "High alert". A few hours later, the fever was back – now in full force spiking at 103 F. He looked very sick and his body was on fire. We put some cold compress and made a quick executive decision to take him to the hospital (Emergency room – this time).

It was his first visit to the emergency room since he was born. As the doctors started to do his intake, we already felt a large disconnect with the providers, since the doctors in the Emergency Department are mostly equipped to deal with acute illness in normally healthy people. Rajan was now officially in the chronic illness category. Although I did not know the term and its implications at the time, I very clearly felt the effects of it. After we went over the history with the doctors, one of them suggested to do a spinal tap to check for possibility of meningitis.

It always amazes me how emergency doctors want to jump to doing a spinal tap, as if it was something as simple and routine as a blood draw before considering other options and doing a thorough review. Based upon our previous experience, we suggested that they take a urine sample instead and refused permission for a spinal tap. We also asked that they contact his surgeon Dr. G and get us moved from the emergency department to the pediatric ward of the hospital as soon as possible, so that he would get more appropriate care as required.

This was not a children's hospital and this was Flint, Michigan. So, any kind of specialty care was not exactly easy to come by. In a couple of hours, we found ourselves admitted into a ward on the pediatric floor of the same hospital – Hospital H. In a way, it was deja vu, but in another sense it felt extremely different. After all, this was the general ward and could hardly be compared with NICU.

This second hospitalization felt like a blur. The one thing I do remember from the hospitalization is that I specifically asked for a discussion with Dr. G after the results of the urine test came in. In our discussion, Dr. G explained the results. Sure enough it was UTI again. I was getting sick of hearing the term and demanded that we have a plan for preventing these infections.

As we battled with controlling the fever and determining next steps, three days passed and we were getting ready to be discharged from the hospital on 28th January. The new plan was not that much different. He was discharged with a new antibiotic that was to be started on the day after the discharge. The new antibiotic was Augmentin (a type of penicillin antibiotic – a combination of amoxicillin and clavulanate potassium). A couple of days later, he developed very loose stools (p.s diarrhea is listed as the #1 potential side effect of this drug). So, this medicine also was not working. What do we do? We had an outpatient appointment with Dr. A (a pediatric infectious disease specialist) two days later.

We explained the side effects to Dr. A and he changed the medicine to Ceftin (a drug in the category of cephalosporins), but we now struggled with severe vomiting (with nausea and vomiting listed under the so called "less serious" side effects). Two days later, we found ourselves in the outpatient clinic of Dr. A along with Dr. G so they could make a plan together. This time, the decision was made to go with Suprax (another cephalosporin antibiotic). As we kept our fingers crossed, we were happy to know that he seemed to tolerate this new antibiotic well (Whew!).

While the general idea is to be off medicines as much as possible, it is somewhat strange to feel happy about being on a medicine that works (or at least does not have serious side effects!). During my discussion with Dr. G, he mentioned that the occurrence of UTIs in patients like Rajan was due to the existence of a fistula connecting the rectum to a part of the urinary tract (the urethra in Rajan's case). This connection in the form of the fistula could be the pathway for bacteria from the gut to make it to the urinary tract and result in a UTI. My obvious question to him was – What should we be doing to keep him safe from UTIs, given the knowledge of the fistula? He responded back with some kind of statistic and about how small this connection can be and how low the occurrence of UTIs was in cases like this.

Frankly, I thought the whole explanation was absolute "BULLSHIT!" Later when I researched this, much to my disgust and anger, it was clearly recommended that anorectal malformation patients with any kind of fistula be placed on an appropriate daily dose of prophylactic antibiotic right after colostomy up to the point that they undergo corrective surgery.

This is a crucial step in care for anorectal malformation patients as they traverse the roadmap of surgical and medical care. Being on the right dose of the prophylactic antibiotic was essential. But we knew little to nothing about these protocols or precautions. It was only now that we felt a feeling of relief in the sense of having determined the appropriate level of protection that he needed to stay infection free. It sure was annoying to realize that much of this agony could have been prevented, had proactive protocol based steps been followed weeks ago.

A moderate amount of stability seemed to have seeped into our lives. This included managing Rajan's ostomy, monitoring his food intake (which fortunately was getting better), keeping him infection free, mostly worrying about short term and long term goals, and keeping my job (from which I had taken a long hiatus) -- - all in that order! As I returned to work, I could feel the tension rising within me when it came to questions from colleagues.

Most people understood the discharge/returning home as the end of a rough first month of life implying that whatever happened, was resolved. With me still fairly naive about all this myself, I didn't bother trying to give any detailed answers about either the condition or the roadmap (what roadmap? I thought to myself) ahead of us. I did take the time to really start digging into information about "anorectal malformations". In the vast majority of google searches, papers published by a surgeon by the name "Dr. Alberto Peña" kept coming up.

I started printing these papers and reading them. The terminology and the base medical knowledge required to appropriately comprehend the papers kept me from getting a good grasp on what to expect. Besides, the papers were written so much from a testing and operating point of view that it didn't help me get a good idea of what I was really looking for – "a roadmap"…something that would guide us as we took this strange and scary journey. Something that would help us interpret the events that would occur as – either part of the planned journey or as unexpected surprises.

One thing became clear, this doctor – Dr. Peña worked in a hospital in Long Island, NY and from his resume and credentials seemed to be not only an expert, but also someone who was very dedicated to this cause. In an upcoming follow up appointment with Dr. G, we took a paper written by Dr. Peña with us. He did his routine examination and asked us about how Rajan was doing. Then, Sheri and I (who had planned and rehearsed our talk) approached the topic with Dr. G. We started by asking him if he was familiar with anyone who would be considered an expert in the field of anorectal malformation related corrective surgeries and its management. We also asked him if he knew about the work of Dr. Peña. Much to our surprise, he was quite familiar with Dr. Peña, his work and his status as an expert in this field. He gladly agreed with our desire to seek advice and treatment from Dr. Peña. While we were getting familiar with Dr. Peña and his amazing work, it was still foreign and distant to us. Dr. G (despite all our reservations about the potential gaps in care that we may have been subject to) was at the end of the day the doctor who would be physically available to help us in the city of Flint, Michigan.

My personal knowledge of children's hospitals in the United States was almost non-existent given my brief experience of seven years living in this country. As we explored the idea of seeking care with Dr. Peña, I realized that I didn't have time to dwell on how uninformed I was or about what kind of impact this doctor's ego might have if we switched our son's care to another doctor that was three states and 720 miles away. While we were convinced that we would seek the best care possible for our son, we also wanted to make sure that immediate appropriate care from the local doctor was not compromised in any way.

The journey into exploring our options started with searching the internet and reading published papers (most links to papers on the internet provided limited access, such as being able to view just the abstract, rather than the full article). Then – what happened can be only best described as divine intervention. In this relatively unknown city of Flint Michigan (which was formerly famous due to proximity to the then automotive capital of the world – Detroit) we had become friends with a family of a couple that happened to be doctors, who had a son that was the same age as Roshan. We had met at a common friend's party and had exchanged numbers and had become close family friends. We had been so busy with learning how to manage Rajan's care that we had not reached out to them to talk about how things had been in the past month. Then Dimple (the wife) called Sheri and invited us to come over to their house for dinner.

It was the first time that we had really ventured out of the house since Rajan was born. We learned that Harkamal (the husband) was visiting home since he was doing his residency in Long Island, NY while his wife and son were in Michigan. Being apart was not easy on the family, but they were managing the situation the best they could. On this particular weekend, he was home and they were enjoying a family reunion.

In a very typical hospitable manner, Harkamal offered me a drink (scotch) as soon as I arrived. I was pretty naïve when it came to my knowledge and choice of alcoholic drinks. With a single person income (Sheri was not working at the time) there was not a whole lot of indulgence in any expensive alcoholic drink other than the simple beer that was affordable.

I accepted the drink, since saying something like "Do you have a beer?" It appeared to be the most ridiculous question to even attempt to ask Harkamal. Harkamal had great taste in scotch: Black label, Red label and Dewars bottles stood in his cellar with very little space for any other alcohol to compete. On that night, I picked "Dewars" since I daringly announced "I'll have what you are having" (having no knowledge of any difference between the alcohols). As I sipped on this smooth drink, I seemed to have another realization – that of "Oh my God… I can't believe I have been missing this experience all my life thus far!" Needless to say, the potent 18% alcohol and my abstinence from it for months made me quite "relaxed" for the first time in a long time. Then the topic came up and Harkamal and Dimple asked more about the condition Rajan had. As Roshan played with their son and as Rajan slept calmly in the busy /loud apartment that we sat in, I started describing Rajan's congenital condition. Only a few minutes into the conversation, Harkamal exclaimed with astonishment and wonder…"Oh Man… you are not going to believe this!!!"

The words anorectal malformation, colorectal surgery and Dr. Peña meant a lot to Harkamal in his situation at the time. Theories about coincidences are just as debatable and intriguing as the phenomenon of coincidences itself. This felt like "divine intervention". As a part of his residency, he had several rotations. His rotation at the time was in the unit of pediatrics – at Children's hospital S and there he was- working with the colorectal surgery team led by none other than the legendary Dr. Alberto Peña! Harkamal was working with Dr. Peña on a daily basis.

As I kept wondering about how in the heck against all odds – this were to happen, Harkamal was very forthright in his recommendation to us. From what he had seen working there for a few months, he recommended that we see Dr. Peña for a consult for a minimum and then take it from there. This was a historic day – it was more than just a get together with our family friends – it was the beginning of the making of history for Rajan and for our family.

CHAPTER 19: GOING TO NEW YORK

I continued educating myself by reading papers on the internet about anorectal malformation (this by exploring every page of google results for the search until they become so dilute that they no longer addressed any true combination of the two words). I requested Harkamal to see if he could set up an appointment with Dr. Peña as soon as possible. With him working with Dr. Peña, we had an obvious advantage in getting an appointment.

As soon as the appointment date was set (March 8th. 2015), I booked my ticket for a one day round trip to New York by Spirit airlines. We had discussed the thought about Sheri and I taking Rajan but decided against it, given how unstable Sheri still felt. Although she wanted to help and do everything she could, we decided that I would take Rajan – our three month old baby by myself on this trip. It was going to be a quick trip – leaving early in the morning that day and returning the next day while staying at Harkamal's apartment for the night. I tried not to think much about my nervousness about taking Rajan by myself on a flight, by letting the "brave" part of my brain win over the "nervous" part.

Before I knew it, the day arrived. Sheri and I woke up early to get ready for the early flight (7:00 am departure) from Detroit (66 miles from Flint). We left at 5:00 am knowing that traffic would be light at that early hour and I was expecting to arrive an hour before departure. Since I did not have any bags to check in, I anticipated this to all flow well. We arrived at the airport at 6:05 am. I placed Rajan in the car seat that I was taking with me on the trip and had a backpack for my overnight clothes, and diapers, meds and clothes for Rajan. I had chosen to take a car seat instead of a stroller since I would need the car seat for travel while in New York. Sheri dropped me off at the departures area and I really did not want her to stay or wait since parking and coming back to the terminal was always a pain at the Detroit airport. As I got out of the car, I grabbed the cell phone and after kissing my wife good bye, entered the departures check in area with car seat with baby in hand and a backpack on my back. For this early in the morning, the departures area looked very busy and loud and caught me by surprise.

Quickly my surprise turned into worry as I realized that there was a long winding line for checking in at the Spirit airlines counter. They had only two check in counters open and running at that time of the day which seemed very inadequate for the number of people who were in line waiting to check in.

I swear I felt a gallon of burning acid secrete in my stomach churning, as it reflected the debilitating restless anxiety in my brain. I looked at my watch. It read 6:20 am and I had barely moved five feet. The counter looked like it was a million miles away and New York felt a lot further than a flight away. The more I thought about how slow the line was progressing, the more anxious I became and the negative thoughts started spiraling out of control in my mind.

What if I didn't make this flight? What if Rajan did not get to see Dr. Peña? What if buying another ticket was going to be a problem? What about getting more time off from my work? What if I lost my job due to taking too many days off? What would happen of my legal status in this country? What would happen to my family?...On and on it went one negative thought sprouting into several negative thoughts as if it were a rapidly progressing viral infection.

It's amazing how a stressful situation can get the mind generating the wildest possible negative thoughts with no regard to the feasibility of them actually happening. I tried to break out of the negative thought cycle and encouraged myself to think about possibilities and maybe even miracles. I was half way through the line which was encouraging, but it was 6:40 am and 20 minutes to departure without having checked in was extremely discouraging. After another agonizing five minutes, I was starting to think that a miracle might still happen because I was only 3 persons away from the counter. But I knew that if the flight was truly going to depart at 7:00 am, I had security to get through and a terminal to get to and there was no way this was going to be humanly possible. But I was hoping against hopes as I approached the counter. I was desperately hoping for the flight to be delayed, so I would have a chance to be on it.

Then the lady at the counter stated in a very sterile voice that the flight was full. "The flight was full? How could that be? I have a confirmed ticket and I am not on the flight yet. So how in the world can this flight be full?"

I yelled back at the lady at the counter. She did not think that my comment and question was worth answering, so she carried on with her work and gave me a blank stare as if my reaction was irrelevant in this situation. "Listen ma'am, I have to be on this flight. It is very important". *Isn't that what every person who is travelling feels?...* I thought to myself. Then the lady was on the phone for a few seconds and after getting off the phone she replied, in the same sterile voice that the gates were closed and that was it.

I was going to miss that flight. Whether the reason was the flight being full or my timing, it did not matter. The gate and aircraft door were closed for departure. Opening the airplane door after the flight is cleared for takeoff, would be a federal offense unless it was for a justifiable emergency. I had an emergency, but it was far from being considered as one by the lady I was standing in front of, let alone a justifiable one.

I told the lady this was a medical emergency and that my son needed to be seen by this doctor in New York later that afternoon. It was imperative that we see him because of his condition and that his future depended on it. She spoke in the same cold tone that I had missed the flight and the only thing she could do is see if I could be rescheduled on another flight. My brain was not processing information in a rational way and after standing in line and being told "flight is full" followed by "doors have closed", I was in full lash out mode and my anger had risen to unprecedented levels. I asked her a rather ridiculous question which could have even being perceived as threatening in some respects.

I said to her "Look here lady, are you going to let me get on that plane with my child or not? The time we are spending arguing about this could have been better used to get me checked in." Then it seems like everything was a blur...In my anger I asked her "Do you have any kids?" She replied "No" to which I responded ... "YOU AND YOUR AIRLINE ARE LIARS AND YOU HAVE NO COMPASSION WHAT SOEVER" I ended up lashing out at this person.

It never struck me that she could have been just the innocent worker in a broken and mismanaged system over which she had little control. But at this moment in time, my brain was not geared to think of all that. I refused to talk with her anymore and without any regard to any damn rules, went across to the next counter and asked about my options for the next available flight.

My heart was beating over 100 beats a minute and adrenaline was flowing like a river inside me. The person at the counter typed away on the computer and then responded that there was another flight available to La Guardia, New York departing at 9:30 am and would get me in New York at 11:15 am. My appointment was at 1:00 pm and I thought...well... maybe this could work after all...So, I got myself and Rajan checked in to the flight departing at 9:30 am.

After going through security, I felt my blood pressure and heart rate slowly come back to normal, although I was still very upset. It was a bit strange for me to get so upset. But, it was perhaps the outpouring of months of frustration, anger and sadness in me that had erupted like a volcano at the Spirit airlines counter.

CHAPTER 20: BABY ON BOARD

I regained my composure and somewhat relaxed my stance and went to the departure gate. It looked rather empty and the state of the carpets and décor inside Detroit airport reflected the economic crisis the city was in. I didn't care about the décor. I felt tired and sat on one of the seats (all of which were ragged and many were ripped). Rajan had been sleeping in his car seat through this whole ordeal. I placed his car seat on the seat beside me and felt relieved to set aside my duffel bag. Since we had only one cell phone, there was no way of contacting Sheri during her drive back to Flint.

So I called about 45 minutes later, told her that I was still at the gate and now waiting for the next flight which was about three hours later. I could tell that she felt worried and helpless being away from me at this time. Rajan then woke up and began crying. I got him out of the car seat and held him in my lap, and fed him a bottle of formula. Although taking care of our baby was no foreign task to me, taking care of Rajan with the history of his condition and in a place away from home and doing it without the help of my wife, made me feel like a nervous dad. Perhaps the delay helped in some ways by calming my nerves to some extent, and getting ready for the journey ahead of us. It was now time to board the plane.

A tiny surge of excitement coursed through my veins. The flight was packed. I checked the car seat at the coat / curb-side check in and got settled in my seat with Rajan in my lap and buckled my seat belt as the pilot made his usual announcement of flight duration and so on. My brain was not attentive to these details as my focus was on getting through the flight and getting to the appointment – which was the objective of this trip and which I was anticipating to be the turning point of care for Rajan.

When you have access to the best care because of proximity to pediatric specialty hospitals, it is hard to imagine what life feels like when you don't have that kind of access. We were in that unfortunate category at the time and I can still remember how it stinks to feel that way.

After caring for Rajan for three months, I had gotten a good feel for how his body worked...well the part that got more attention than it would have normally gotten for any baby was of course his GI tract. It's quite interesting to note that the word "GI" consists of the word "gastro" – meaning to do with gasses. We don't tend to think much of this word, much like we don't think much of our human systems functionality when we are healthy and feeling good. But the creation and release of gasses is a very important aspect of the functionality of the defecation system – as important as the evacuation of feces itself.

The products of the bowels – the things that help in us feeling relieved and vibrant – the things that we avoid talking about in our day to day conversations – stools – had become the center of our attention in terms of care for Rajan at this time. Half way through the flight, I sensed that his colostomy bag was full and bloated. The good news about a bloated colostomy bag is that it is doing its job and that there are no leaks...which is why the trapped gasses are keeping the bag bloated. You can very well imagine what a fully bloated bag implies.... Not a good situation. The bad news – it needs to be relieved...and relieved soon, else we face the consequences of bad foul odor.

It suddenly struck me – I was surrounded by people in a packed flight on the economy class and this kind of accident (which is no big deal at home) would be a disaster to deal with in public. Normally, when the bag is filled only with gasses, we would vent the bag when at home...but now I was not at home and venting in the plane while being packed like sardines on that flight was NOT going to be a good idea.

I hoped desperately that there was a bathroom on the plane…since it was not a very big plane. Fortunately, there was one. I took him to the tiny airplane bathroom, pulled down the child seat, laid him down, and vented the gas. When you take care of your own child, it is a completely different feeling. Nothing is too bad or terrible to do – when it means safety and well-being of your child. After our business was done, I felt as relieved as his colostomy bag did!

Every little aisle and every tight space with the baby in my arms felt a lot smaller and tighter than it had ever seemed before. I nestled back into my seat with Rajan in my lap. He was a good baby through the flight thus far and I hoped for that to continue. While I had a brief 10 to 15 minute nap on the flight, Rajan slept as the airplane engines hummed away. I was now hoping for the announcement for the flight to land, but instead I heard an altogether different announcement that grabbed my attention.

The pilot announced that there was severe weather in New York and that the decision to either go to a different airport or to circle in the air around the same airport was being evaluated. Both options felt like a slap in my face after the mis-adventure I had in the morning of having missed my original flight. A few nervous minutes passed by and then the pilot was back on the speaker system.

All passengers seemed to have sighed after he announced that the plane was after all going to land at La Guardia. When we landed, it became clear to us what the pilot had meant when he mentioned "severe weather". The ground was all "white" covered with what looked like a good 2 to 3 inches of snow. Additionally, snow was blowing all over the place making visibility a big challenge. I was actually surprised how they made the decision to land at this airport. With these conditions, I anticipated that flights had started to be delayed or cancelled as we taxied to our terminal. The taxiing took a good 25 minutes and I imagined what a mess the traffic control office might have been at this time. Getting off the airplane was undoubtedly a challenge I was not expecting. But then again, ordinary experiences of everyday life did not seem to the norm in those days of our lives. I got a real feel for what New York crowds in a crowded plane that has been delayed looks and acts like! They were agitated, ruthless and rude and didn't give a damn about a dad carrying a baby.

I wasn't looking for special treatment, but sure as heck did not appreciate the shoving and nudging to get to the front of the plane in a hurry and stares that I got when I was trying to gather all the stuff for Rajan. I am sure everyone had a reason for why they were in a hurry. However, I doubt that there was anyone else on that plane who was carrying a baby with a congenital defect whose initial treatment had gone real shitty, who had missed the first flight and was not even sure if he could keep the appointment with this surgeon, since the circumstances were making this more and more of a seemingly impossible task.

CHAPTER 21: SNOWY TOUCHDOWN

After much disgust with the airplane crowd, I stepped out of the plane with my duffel bag and Rajan situated back in his car seat. I regretted not carrying a backpack instead of the duffel bag because of the cumbersome feeling of carrying the duffel bag in one hand and the car seat in the other. I turned on my cell phone immediately and noticed there were voice messages from Sheri and my friend Harkamal. I called Sheri first to let her know that I had arrived but chose not go into details of the flight or about the weather.

Next I called Harkamal and he said he was there waiting at the baggage claim / passenger exit area. Carrying a duffel bag in one hand and a baby in a car seat in another is not as easy as I thought it would be – a realization that hit me after walking for about 10 minutes while approaching the baggage claim area. Everything at the airport looked so busy. I was used to a fair amount of domestic and international travel, but everything seemed amplified at this time. Then I saw Harkamal waving to me.

He was calling out my name, but in the noise I didn't hear him, but rather saw him first. Harkamal had drove around the airport since you can't park by the passenger pick up area and he did not want to park in the airport long term parking since that would have meant even more delays in getting out of there. I placed the car seat with Rajan in the back seat and bucked him in. Harkamal drove an old fairly beat up Chevy minivan. An odd choice for a man of his tastes.

Soon I realized that his BMW X5 was back home in Michigan. Having the van with him in New York had another reason that he would go on to tell me later. As Harkamal started driving, I asked if we could still make the appointment with Dr. Peña.

Harkamal had managed to push the appointment time out, but with the delay in arriving at New York, the weather and the traffic, we would not get there before 4:00 pm - well over 2 hours past the original appointment time. He told me in a calm voice that the visit with Dr. Peña was not going to happen on that day. I felt sick and angry and irritated about not having made it and my thoughts went back to the long line at Detroit, the missed flight, the plane journey, the bathroom incident and the duffel bag / car seat challenge.

All this was not going well. I asked if we could see Dr. Peña the next day and he replied stating that he would work something out. "Work something?" I thought... and what if he is not able to work something out? I didn't say anything because nothing coming out of my mouth after just about everything going wrong was going to come out right. So I nodded and said "OK". Beggars can't be choosers, especially beggars who haven't even arrived on time.

As evening approached, the anxiety and excitement calmed down to the point where I was able to actually have a conversation with Harkamal and even soak in the new surroundings and city that I had never visited before. I was in New York – Yeah! Harkamal took us to the place he was living in. It was the basement of a house that he along with a couple of roommates had rented. It wasn't in the best of conditions – but hey these guys were living like single people and they were all away from home and with the busy / ridiculous demands of them being residents of LIJ (Long Island Jewish) hospital, keeping their home tidy was "non-existent" on their list of things to do. I didn't mind it one bit and it took me back to my good old college days where keeping the place nice and tidy was the last thing a guy would do, even if he did have the time to do it! Harkamal made some phone calls and it was a pleasure to listen to him talk in "Hindi" as they made plans for dinner.

Of course, we went to an Indian restaurant. I felt a bit strange carrying our little baby in a car seat instead of a stroller, while I was in the company of what looked like single guys (although most of them were not). I didn't care as much about what food I ordered; it was the strong drink I was really looking forward to that night. I am not sure if it was the drink or my mental belief in the benefit of the drink in calming my nerves – but the single drink and the good old Indian food and its aromas made me relaxed.

Despite all the difficulties, I had many things to be thankful for – I was in New York with Rajan and the prospect of having Dr. Peña see him the next day was decent and that made me feel content. I was also thankful for sitting in the backseat of the van and not driving since I was exhausted from the stress of the day. I may have taken a small nap while I sat in the back seat with Rajan as I stared out of the window while watching the lights of Long Island go by. One of Harkamal's friends was out of town and they let me use his twin bed to sleep in for the night.

CHAPTER 22: THE APPOINTMENT

I woke up the next morning and felt all the anxiety and excitement return into my system. Whatever this day was going to bring me, I was ready. I was not thinking of anything other than just making the much anticipated appointment happen. Harkamal left early in the morning and told me that he would call me once he got an appointment with Dr. Peña and then would come and pick me up from his home.

I waited and waited and kept looking at my phone all morning. Then all of a sudden the phone rang and it was him. Harkamal was brief. He said he was on his way and we were to meet Dr. Peña in one hour. Fortunately, Harkamal lived close to the hospital (10 minute ride). In less than half hour of his phone call, Harkamal had brought Rajan and me to the second floor of a building. He asked me to stay put and assured me that he would be back with Dr. Peña. He worked his magic and soon I realized this was not the typical appointment. It was a consult that Dr. Peña had agreed to - with the bare minimum EHR (Electronic Health Record) system inclusions that would allow us to get testing done along with the brief visit.

Just before meeting Dr. Peña, I had snuck in the bathroom and deflated the bag, just in case things were going to take a while with the meeting and with testing that might follow. By this time, Sheri and I were quite attuned to Rajan's modified anatomy and the two additional stomas felt much less foreign to us than they did initially.

I could sense things like "it's been several hours (time to deflate bag) or after several hours the bag is not even slightly inflated – something's not quite right – is there a leak due to improper adhesion of the bag to the skin? We had also become experts in caring for the skin surrounding the stoma that was especially vulnerable to rashes due to an unusually larger potential for exposure to stool or sometimes due to constantly being exposed to the adhesive materials of the bag.

Then the moment arrived. Dr. Peña appeared with Harkamal. He was a tall lanky man with glasses, wearing his bright white doctor's coat. There was an unmistakable air of authority and confidence he exuded. He introduced himself and greeted me with "Hello Mr. Dahale"– another very characteristic formal mannerism of Dr. Peña that made him unique. He greeted me with a hand shake which was a bit unexpected in terms of it not being as firm as I was expecting it to be. He had long hands and a medium grip hand shake. Perhaps he was such a perfectionist that he saved dexterity of his hands for what mattered most to him – precision, accuracy and an uncanny artistic ability in performing one of the most sacred revered acts of medicine in humanity – SURGERY. After I introduced myself, Dr. Peña asked me Rajan's history. I described it with an average amount of medical savviness and a decent amount of the experience of observing and caring for him at home. Then Dr. Peña examined Rajan.

The first thing that caught his eye, was a long transverse scar running across his abdomen. He looked at the two stomas and carefully evaluated the distance between them (one of the visual markers and predictors of the success of potential future surgeries and ultimately prognosis of the eventual functional outcome. Then he looked at me and asked me "What is this scar from?" pointing to the long and thick scar running several inches across his abdomen.

Dr. Peña was incredibly smart and intuitive, yet never assuming. When I mentioned about the scar being from his colostomy surgery, his expressions said it all. Over the years, he had developed a way to comment on the work of other surgeons in an unpretentiously honest manner without being disrespectful. In this case, he mentioned about the scar being longer than necessary and cosmetically inadequate. With that said, he asked if there were any functional issues with the colostomy. I mentioned about the mucous fistula prolapse incident a few days after the colostomy creation surgery and that things were "well" except for battling with infections and finding the right antibiotic.

Then, Dr. Peña did a physical exam of Rajan. He was primarily interested in seeing how his perineum looked like. The appearance of the perineum is one of the several indicators of prognosis of bowel control (the primary functional outcome in all anorectal malformations). Dr. Peña ordered a distal colostogram to be performed in half hour.

The physical exam, my narrative and the distal colostogram would be the three critical pieces of information he used to determine the course of action. Yes, Dr. Peña had thousands of cases of experience to be able to be definitive about course of action to take for each patient, but his unique quality was that he treated every essential component of decision making with great respect and never took things for granted. Before long, we were in the radiology room.

As I waited with Rajan in the room for a few minutes, Dr. Peña and another doctor came in along with a radiology technician. Then something strange happened.

Dr. Peña took the lead in terms of observing and giving detailed instructions to the technician performing the procedure. *The procedure requires a dye to be inserted into the mucous fistula – the fistula that connects to the distal end of the colon. It is incredibly important to conduct this procedure correctly. Doing the procedure incorrectly leads to the wrong conclusions being drawn about the anatomy of the colon, which in turn leads to the wrong type of surgery selection and/or realization of the true anatomy while operating as opposed to knowing the anatomy before operating.*

An incorrectly conducted colostogram is the equivalent of doing a blind or an ill-informed surgery. The pressure of the inserted dye must be adjusted and made sufficient enough to help determine the true end point of the distal colon. The position of this "true end point" and its distance from the perineum informs the choice of surgery type and also of the surgical approach. Amazingly, this critical piece of information helps determine (calculate) a critical parameter called sacral ratio. This ratio along with surgical skill determine the prognosis of bowel control for the child – Incredible!

I watched and waited as the professionals in white clothing did their thing. I watched in awe as a large syringe with a pre-mixed dye was injected through the mucous fistula using a tube connected to the syringe. A real time display of an ultrasound was used and x rays were ready to be deployed. The live display enabled the team to get the dye injected with the appropriate pressure until the true "end" of the distal colon was perceived and seen on the images.

Pictures were then taken to capture the anatomy. This process took a few iterations and adjustments – all done under the guidance of Dr. Peña until he was convinced that the tube and the dye had reached the appropriate end. *This end of the colon in most malformations terminated in the form of a fistula connecting to some point on the urinary tract. The relative location of his fistula and its proximity to organs helps determine the name of the fistula and also the malformation.*

The images were taken and Dr. Peña was satisfied with how they looked on the monitor. This "live" imaging was impressive to me and made me realize the importance of timeliness of the results in the "quality" of imaging. Also, it was unusual and interesting for me to see how much Dr. Peña was personally involved in the imaging process – given that he was an extremely busy surgeon (isn't every surgeon in the world extremely busy?). I didn't know what to expect next. Just like that Dr. Peña said thanks and left the room. I left the room with Rajan shortly after getting him dressed.

Next, I met with Harkamal, who then advised me that Dr. Peña had to leave to go out of the country that evening. Based upon Harkamal's request, he had made time to see Rajan in what would technically be considered an unscheduled visit/encounter. I was extremely grateful for Dr. Peña taking the time to see Rajan. A few minutes after the visit, I met with Dr. Peña in his office. Dr. Peña had made his diagnosis after reviewing the test results and the physical examination of the perineum. He had calculated Rajan's sacral ratio and based upon his anatomy, classified him as a prostatic fistula patient. He had also prophesied his prognosis as having a 60% chance of bowel control.

I had been a fairly "numbers and statistics" savvy guy especially since I had completed my master's degree in industrial engineering with a focus on quality and reliability – a sub specialty that involved an emphasis on an in-depth study of applied statistics. In order to do this, I had taken some pure statistics classes and several advanced engineering classes. I had moderately enjoyed the statistics class but greatly enjoyed the quality engineering classes where we actually got to apply the concepts to solve real problems.

I tried to digest this piece of statistical information and it really felt like a very difficult task – mostly because digesting something like this for your own son is a lot harder to do than doing it for someone else, but also because statistics like these do need explanation in terms of what they "really" mean. They are well understood by clinicians or surgeons but rarely understood by patients and families in terms of their true implications.

The number 60% was lodged in my head for ever. It stood for the probability of an outcome for something we (lucky healthy people) take for granted. The daunting part of the number of course was its complement – for every percentage of probability of success is the probability of failure. Now there was the question of which side of the fence Rajan would eventually be on – the 40% which never ended up having bowel control or the 60% that would. It is hard to explain the mind games statistics play in real scenarios in terms of their emotional impact on patients and families since all we want is for our child to be healthy and OK and no other percentage describing anything else matters mostly because rational thinking takes a back seat in situations like these.

CHAPTER 23: MOVING FORWARD

Dr. Peña then advised me to work with his trusted nurse –Cathy, to decide on the logistics of the next surgery to correct this problem, if we chose to pursue Rajan's treatment with him and the hospital he worked for. My interaction with Cathy led me to see her in her office. In the hallways and in her office there were many "kid friendly" cartoon caricatures and also some pictures of multi-colored fish. I remembered seeing a small pin in the form of this fish pinned to Dr. Peña's white coat earlier that day.

Since the fish had peaked my attention and curiosity, I asked about what the multi-colored fish meant. Cathy went on to describe the fish to be a "rainbow fish" and it significance to be in the form of Dr. Peña whose life and work was analogous to the story of the rainbow fish where the fish gives away a color to each fish he sees. Similar to the story, Dr. Peña believed in always teaching his learning and skills to other doctors and nurses and to brighten the lives of the children he touched, by giving them the "color" they lacked.

Cathy logged into her computer and after accessing Dr. Peña's surgery schedule, remarked "I have the first available open slot for May 3rd. 2005 in the morning at 7:30 am. Would you like to take it?". It was interesting for me to note that our conversation and interactions had gone in the last few hours, from a consult to booking a date for surgery quite rapidly.

From the multitude of patients that Cathy had seen, perhaps it was quite clear to her that most patients / families with children with anorectal malformations chose to come to Dr. Peña for surgery after initially consulting with him. It was sort of a "no brainer" in the vast majority of cases. I didn't want to lose the spot on his calendar, so replied saying "Yes, I would like to take that slot, but would like to check with my family and hope that we will still be able to reschedule in case of the unlikely event that the particular date did not work". Cathy replied back by saying that this decision was more to do with putting a placeholder and that the final confirmation of dates would happen after several other formal steps including insurance approvals, etc. were in place and including confirming our decision to work with Dr Peña for operating on Rajan. This reassurance from Cathy and the time period between March and May to confirm things, put my mind at ease. It also automatically created the rough sketch of a path in my mind for Rajan's roadmap that did not exist before.

Soon after my conversation with Cathy, I called Sheri and told her about my interaction with Dr. Peña and his team and that I definitely felt the future course of Rajan's treatment to be with him, and also that we had a potential date for the next surgery. I was expecting Sheri to be a bit surprised about already discussing the date for surgery. But she was not surprised, rather elated to hear the formation of a concrete step forward in the right direction for Rajan.

I heard her mention the date of surgery to Mavshi in the background, who in turn instinctively checked out what day May 3rd. fell on – It was a Tuesday. Mavshi quickly reaffirmed that it would be good and auspicious for the surgery to happen on a Tuesday since it aligned with the day of worship for our family goddess. "This day will be blessed for Rajan", Mavshi muttered in the background. The series of discussions I had with the doctors, nurses and my family seemed to keep building my confidence in the creation of a good solid plan for Rajan.

As I hung up the phone after my conversation with Sheri and Mavshi, I felt a strange feeling. It's hard to describe the feeling, but it was akin to the feeling experienced when some much needed nutritious food makes its way to a starved hungry belly. A feeling of the filling up of the bucket of hope and reassurance. The stress, and the worry and the uncertainty had not diminished, yet for a few minutes, I was able to switch myself form the mode of the "anxious and worried dad" to the "encouraged and hopeful dad".

All said and done, the monumental event of being seen by Dr. Peña, for which I had flown to New York, had finally materialized despite all odds. Little did I know that life ahead was going to be filled with struggles like these in the journey of chronic care, even while living in a country with such abundant resources. It was really the beginning phases of the "bumpy road" that Dr. G had described.

There are generally two types of approaches people develop when they realize they are on a bumpy road – a) they get off it (avoidance) or b) they learn to navigate it (continuous adaptation). For us, option "a" was never going to work for many reasons. Life had already taught me that option "b" will be much harder in terms of energy required to traverse it and patience and resilience required to sustain it, but worth it in the end. So I took a deep breath as I chose option "b" in my head. I finally had a chance to remember that Harkamal had wanted to tell me something important when I had arrived in New York.

I turned my attention to my good friend, and asked him what it was that he had meant to tell me. Also, I needed to discuss about my options to return back to Michigan, since I had missed by flight the previous day – this time consciously. Harkamal went on to tell me the shocking news of his decision to quit the residency program at LIJ and to resume it elsewhere – most likely closer to Michigan, and his family, while focusing in an area that was less demanding than surgery. This decision of course was deliberated and discussed between him and his wife over a long period of time before it became final. The culmination of this decision making was in the form of his "last day" at LIJ being today.

"WOW! I thought to myself – how fortunate I was to have this visit with Dr. Peña". I felt an overwhelming amount of gratitude for Harkamal for all he had done thus far. Harkamal then went on to inform me that he was packing up his stuff and driving back to Michigan in his van and that I had a choice of helping him and giving him company driving back – OR – to book a flight back from New York. My last experience at La Guardia airport and the desire to pay back Harkamal instantly drove me to decide on helping him pack and drive back with him in his van.

Luckily Harkamal had either already taken much of his stuff back, or left some things for his buddies, but there really was not a whole lot of things to pack and much of it was consolidated into two large open cardboard boxes that I helped him carry to the van. He chose the good old way of stuffing his clothes into a few large garbage bags. The weather in New Yok was way more pleasant compared to the snow storm the earlier day.

It was sunny and the snow was rapidly melting away and we were about to start our journey to Michigan. It was late afternoon and I thought we would get on the expressway to Michigan right away. But we took a little detour as Harkamal wanted to meet up with some of his friends in Queens, NY. So there were we were – in Queens parked in front of an apartment. I chose to stay back with Rajan in the van as Harkamal went to talk to his friends on the third floor of the apartment complex.

From whatever intuition my "New York naïve" brain experienced, I chose to lock the doors of the van as a gesture of safety and protection in what looked like an uninviting neighborhood. I waited patiently and squished any further thoughts of judging the neighborhood – simply because I knew very little about this place. In about 15 minutes or so (which seemed like eternity), Harkamal returned and we were on our way ... to the next stop – a gas station.

It appeared like a rather unusual gas station since there was an attendant who was filling gas for customers. This was certainly something I was not expecting to see in New York in the year 2005, knowing that "self-serve" had been the norm for the last several years. Harkamal went on to mention that the optional service was offered to customers in the form of this attendant who would not only fill gas but also wipe / clean the windshield if you would like for a small fee. It was also a way for some gas station owners to employ folks who were in much need of making some extra cash to make ends meet. It was quite common to see this type of role being done by an immigrant. This matched the scenarios I was seeing in terms of an Indian guy working as an attendant in the gas station owned by an Indian as well. Harkamal spoke in his native tongue (Punjabi) to thank him and gave him a tip.

We drove only a couple of blocks before Harkamal pointed to a famous Indian sweet / snack store. He said they have the "best samosas" there and asked if we should stop and buy some. I responded "Yes, why not?" With that, he went in and returned with a brown paper bag filled with six samosas whose aroma instantly awoke some hunger in me.

Harmamal and I decided to indulge in eating two samosas each. He folded the ends of the bag with two remaining samosas stating that he was saving those for his wife. With two Samosas in bag, a full tank of gas, a sleeping baby in the car seat and the back of the van loaded with clothes, Harkamal and I set off on the expressway headed west.

CHAPTER 24: THE ROAD TRIP

Getting through New York was as you would expect it to be – very busy and soon after, we were cruising through the long narrow state of Pennsylvania. Harkamal and I talked for the first half hour or so, then we just let music on the radio or some Punjabi songs on CD fill the air in the van. Rajan was sound asleep as we were driving. After a couple of hours, I instinctively reached for his colostomy bag by feeling it over his clothes and realized the bulge.

Since we were not anywhere close to a rest stop, I pre-warned Harkamal that I was about to vent the bag. As an intervention, I opened the window of the rear passenger side just slightly to air out the unpleasant trapped methane. It always made me wonder how such a little baby could produce such a strong odor! Opening the window for a few minutes also provided the opportunity to be refreshed by the cool winter breeze. It had turned dark and we had not really had a proper lunch. Obviously, we were hungry. As we drove, we noticed an exit with the standard fast food restaurants sign coming up. We debated if we should take the exit and with the exit approaching so quickly, decided to take the next food exit. In retrospect, every decision we make – seemingly simple, has consequences.

The consequences, just like the decisions can be ordinary or major. We cruised for another two or three miles past the exit, only to be met with vehicles coming to a rapid halt and to add to that, it looked like a long line of tail lights – all at a standstill! We came to a screeching halt from 70 miles per hour – a few miles past our last opportunity to have had dinner. However, we were in the middle of nowhere in Pennsylvania. It was a dark still chilly night and light snow kept falling off and on. Ok, we were in a traffic jam. So what?

Should clear up soon...right? The rhetorical question remained unanswered after 30 minutes of no movement.

We were getting impatient just sitting in the van and decided to venture out of the van to see if there was any movement in traffic at all. Harkamal and I took turns stepping out into the cold exterior, each of us coming up with the same conclusion – miles of stopped cars and trucks ahead of and behind us and no sign of any movement.

We were trapped, we were immobilized and we were hungry! Also, our van's location in the long traffic jam happened to be high up on somewhat of a cliff. After a long nap, Rajan woke up hungry and I fed him a bottle of prepared milk I had brought with me in the van. Then our own hunger pangs were getting stronger and the "traffic jam induced" anxiety seemed to make the hunger feel worse than normal. It was more than an hour into the traffic jam standstill.

We joked about whether there was enough baby food that we may have to dip into. Then it struck him... the two remaining samosas! Harkamal said a mental silent "sorry" to his wife and we dug into the samosas savoring them as if they were the last piece of food on the earth... actually they were in our van! The gas tank was almost half full...Good, at least we didn't have to worry about freezing in the middle of a traffic jam as long as our car continued to idle and provide us with the much needed warmth.

It was a noisy environment with cars, trucks and busses – all in the mix of the traffic jam helplessly idling away their gas or diesel engines and staying warm in the cold winter night...waiting for the traffic jam to clear. As all the people helplessly waited, most didn't know what had happened. Almost everyone guessed it was an accident but no one could tell how long it was going to take to get traffic flowing again.

Then there was some news that was spreading between people waiting in the jam and we caught wind of it in the occasional "stepping out the van to see if anything ahead of us was moving at all" episodes. The rumor was that a semi carrying gas or some flammable liquid had rolled over and the haz-mat (hazardous materials) control team had to do a complete clean up before anyone could move. The rumor made sense but now we were pushing past the two and half hours of being in a standstill.

It was also a time for other urban legend stories / theories to be told and Harkamal told me one such theory. He said that he had heard that if traffic jams last more than two hours, there is a decent chance that someone in the middle of the line of waiting traffic falls asleep and further delays the traffic jam indefinitely although the jam in front of that person is cleared. Based upon this theory, we were definitely at risk and after hearing that, my frequency of "taking a peek" at the line ahead automatically increased. Time seems to appear to pass very differently in such situations.

The mind tends to be pre-occupied with anxiety, fear, anger, and irritation and all this is supplemented typically by thoughts about the consequences of the delay as well as all the things you could have been doing if you were NOT at a standstill. Rarely do we tend to think of what ELSE we COULD be doing while we are not able to drive. It was perhaps somewhere around the three hour mark, that the traffic finally started moving from the absolute stillness that had preceded for what seemed like an eternity and just like that... vehicles small and big overcame their forced inertia and the much desired "movement" took over.

Such situations are also realizations of appreciation for what our vehicles do for us. The simple fact of our personal transportation vehicles being able to transport us over hundreds of miles turns from something we take for granted to becoming a "real" aspect of appreciation even if it is for just a few moments.

In retrospect, I look back at the incident of the traffic jam and several other situations that followed and wondered about what ELSE I could have done with my mind when the "desired outcome" is primarily led by people or factors completely outside of your control and one important idea came to my mind – "Prayer". *It doesn't matter whom you pray to or how you pray, just the act of doing so channels the mind from the multitrack emotion filled status to a singular track and is typically associated with an automatic "calmness" as you try to get through the difficult situation. Whether such an act influences the actual outcome, can be debatable and ends up being a personal preference. When it comes to choices in such situations, you could spend your time filled with anger, helplessness and despair or in hope and calmness.*

The anticipated 9 to 10 hour journey was now significantly delayed and we had no idea of what else lay ahead of us. The remainder of the journey through the long state of Pennsylvania was uneventful. Soon, we were crossing borders and into the state of Ohio – accompanied by a sense of accomplishment of getting closer to our destination. Only a few miles into the drive and everything started to look blurry. The weather had turned worse and the air was filled with large snowflakes – a great wonder and beauty of nature – but one we couldn't appreciate at this time.

We quickly realized that we were in the "snow belt" of Ohio. We slowed down to protect ourselves from sliding off the expressway and to help us actually see whatever visibility the falling snowflakes and our old Chevy van's headlights would allow. While we had largely become impervious to what time it exactly was, looking at the clock we realized that it was close to 3:00 am.

Fatigue, low visibility and the slow speed and progress toward our destination finally made their impact on our decision making and we decided to take the next exit and pulled over into an empty but well- lit gas station. As the van came to a halt, we finally let our minds and bodies rest and take a much desired nap after the crazy part of the journey we had endured. As the van with its (thankfully) large gas tank idled, I desperately hoped for Rajan to continue to sleep for just a little longer and let me take this much needed nap. My prayer was answered and Harkamal and I reclined the driver and passenger seats and slept for a good hour and half while enjoying the unbuckled feeling.

When we woke up, I offered to drive, but Harkamal did not feel comfortable taking care of Rajan, so he continued to drive for the rest of the journey as well. After having rested, we took our own bathroom breaks at the gas station, refueled the vehicle and felt the distinct optimistic and confident feeling of completing the rest of the journey in "good" time.

The rate of snowfall dropped and the sun was coming out and everything seemed better as the morning showed us promise of getting to our destination that day. We cruised along, took an exit to grab brunch and after approximately five hours of almost non-stop driving, crossed the state of Ohio and half of Michigan to arrive "HOME".

Harkamal dropped Rajan and me off at our house. As I carried Rajan in the car seat up the driveway, we were welcomed by Sheri and Mavshi, for whom it was as much of a relief to see us as it was for me to be home. I handed over our precious cargo "Rajan" to Sheri and she held him close giving him and me kisses as we entered the house.

It was one thing to endure a tough journey, but it was another to do so with a baby and one with colostomy needs. I felt a huge relief in terms of having got through and done "well" with taking care of Rajan – something I was quite nervous about when I had started the journey. As I stood in the shower and let the warm water wash away my built up stress, I reflected on the sequence of events:

Preparing to go to New York →Missed flight →Delayed arrival at New York due to snow storm → Missed appointment with Dr. Peña → Staying at Harkamal and his buddies bachelor pad →Appointment with Dr. Peña → Receiving a prognosis report card for Rajan → Scheduling of his next surgery in Long Island, NY → Missed flight back home → Adventurous ride in Harkamal's van.

Then I breathed a long sigh of relief and rejoiced the simple fact that Rajan and I were back at home and concluded that we had a "successful" trip. Perhaps with every milestone we crossed, our capability to successfully deal with the "long bumpy road" seem to incrementally improve. Rajan's journey had become as much of our family's journey as it was his own. We were glad to be together as a family for the next few months.

CHAPTER 25: GOODBYE

With Mavshi's scheduled departure date arriving soon, we realized how much we had going on, and how essential it was to have the support Mavshi was offering to us in these difficult times. The next important thing to do was to call the airline and change (extend) the departure date for Mavshi. For the next month, Mavshi continued to help us in all possible ways, as we developed a new routine that involved taking care of Rajan and his medical needs along with the basic essentials of our personal and professional lives. With tears in our eyes, and deep appreciation and love for all that Mavshi had done for us, we waved goodbye to each other, as we watched her walk past the security check point into the airport.

CHAPTER 26: PREPARING FOR THE NEXT SURGERY

A few weeks before the scheduled surgery in May, we received a call from Children's Hospital S confirming the surgery date and reminding us of the reality of dealing with more medical care and management that was ahead of us. The call was as essential and informative as it was scary. The conflicting feelings of wanting this surgery (maximizing his chances for the best potential outcome) and not wanting any more surgeries ever (parental wishful thinking) played a tug of war in my brain.

This time around, we planned a different arrangement for Roshan for the time we were going to be away for Rajan's surgery in the month of May in New York. We attempted to request Sheri's mom and sister to help out with watching Roshan as while we were going to be away. Our request for help was met with somewhat of an acknowledgement – so we accepted it knowing that not everyone was going to have an enthusiastic response to taking on additional responsibility. Time flew by and the day was here.

We locked up the house and got into my white Chevy Malibu that was going to help us get to our destination. We first all drove to Sheri's mom's place and dropped off Roshan. We left their house in tears as it felt horrible leaving our three year old for what seemed like an indeterminate amount of time. Perhaps we heard them say Good luck – and maybe we didn't – because we were so engulfed in our anxiety of a major surgery and the worry of leaving our three year old son behind in Michigan.

Sheri and I hugged Roshan multiple times – assuring him that he could call us anytime and we would be there for him – telling him how brave he was – for agreeing to stay back in Michigan without mama and baba. We also assured him that we would be calling him at least twice a day, if not more – and especially before he went to bed to wish him good night.

CHAPTER 27: ON THE ROAD AGAIN

The next thing I knew, we were on the expressway driving to New York State. The bright late spring day was in contrast to the dreary snowy day that I remembered driving back from New York from the previous time in March. The bright rays of the sun seemed to infuse the much needed warmth and energy we aspired, to take on the challenge ahead of us. About half way through our journey, the cell phone rang and it was Ronald McDonald House of Long Island NY calling us to confirm our arrival date and time as well as letting us know that a room was available for us when we would arrive at the "House".

Our journey was pleasantly uneventful and didn't seem as long. Our minds were preoccupied with what was to follow and the miles, minutes and hours just flew by as we cruised through the "not so busy" expressway through the long state of Pennsylvania and into the Empire State. Sheri took care of Rajan through the whole journey and Rajan seemed to enjoy the long ride without being fussy. He napped for most of the day. He was nestled in his car seat and woke up only when he was hungry. Unlike the two star service he received when I managed the limited supplies of bottle milk on the cursed snow storm journey from New York to Michigan in March, Rajan must have enjoyed the five star service of his mama attending to his needs and showering lots of added love, care and attention in the limousine like ride to New York.

By late afternoon, we had successfully navigated New York traffic, staying on the outskirts of New York City and effectively using the paper Atlas map (considered an antiquated concept in today's generation – given the advent of GPS navigation systems and Google maps in recent years).

CHAPTER 28: HOME AWAY FROM HOME

We were warmly greeted by the manager of Ronald McDonald house of Long Island, NY after we entered the premises of the House. This was our first exposure to the operations of the Ronald McDonald House and we were truly humbled by the warmth and generosity of the staff – many of whom were volunteers – donating their time and effort to help strangers like us experience a home away from home during our time of one of the most profound needs of life. I silently resolved to provide the same service to others as a way to pay it forward. The seeds of volunteering at a Ronald McDonald House were planted in my brain. The time would come, when I would fulfil my own promise of giving back to the House.

Ronald McDonald houses: A little history about Ronald McDonald House – It all began in 1974, when three-year-old Kim Hill, the daughter of Philadelphia Eagles football player Fred Hill and his wife, Fran, was being treated for leukemia at St. Christopher's Hospital for Children. Families who travelled far distances seeking treatment at children's hospitals struggled as accommodation in hotels was often unaffordable and inconvenient when it came to the often indeterminate length of stay that would be required for care of their children. Seeing the plight of the children and families, Fran and his wife decided to do something about this and raised money with his colleagues to start a charity that would build "houses" near children's hospitals so that families could have a safe, comfortable and affordable place to stay during the time that the child is undergoing treatment at the hospital.

His vision was supported by Dr. Audrey Evans, the head of the pediatric oncology unit at the Children's Hospital of Philadelphia and later by Don Tuckerman from the

McDonald's advertising agency and thus was born the first Ronald McDonald House in 1974 in Philadelphia. The Ronald McDonald House is often referred to as the "house that love built". Today, more than 250 Ronald McDonald Houses in 26 countries support families around the world – providing comfort to more than 10 million families since 1974.

Every house has bedrooms that are offered to guests which have basic amenities like two beds, a bathroom, toiletries, etc. There is also a common kitchen shared by guests where you can cook your own food if you like. Refrigerator space is provided to each guest and whatever you can fit into two basket containers can be stored in the fridge as yours. Another fridge is labelled "community" fridge and contains items that can be accessed by all guests.

As guests, you can contribute to the community fridge if you would like to. Basic necessities such as milk and cheese are always available in this fridge. There is also a community pantry which houses things such as bread and cereal and a variety of canned and boxed food.

We were given a brief tour of the house and led to our small, cozy and comfortable bedroom. The room was very clean and everything was neatly arranged. One important rule of the house is that every bedroom must be occupied by at least one adult each night that the guest / family stays at the house. Initially this sounds like an inconsiderate rule. But if you think about it for a while, it makes a lot of sense and has a lot of meaning behind it. When your child is in the hospital, parents may often stretch themselves to the max. and tend to not take care of themselves because they feel an overwhelming desire to take care of their child in whatever way they can and taking care of themselves feels selfish and guilt-ridden.

Such a rule forces at least one parent to stay the night at the house while the other parent can stay with the child in *the hospital. This assures that at least one parent is likely to get somewhat of a decent sleep and hence can swap places with the other parent during the day. Of course – the House made exceptions for cases where only one parent was available, if only a single parent was taking care of the child.*

We quickly made our arrangement and being the night owl that I was, I offered to stay at the hospital and Sheri agreed to sleep at the House and come in early in the morning to the hospital. After the long drive, we were happy to retire for the day in our cozy beds and Rajan in a crib they provided. The next day, we were to get Rajan admitted into the hospital. We had little idea about children's hospitals since the hospital in Flint Michigan was really an adult hospital with a pediatric ward. Children's Hospital S– in a way was really not that different, except that it was much bigger and happened to have the world's best pediatric colorectal surgeon working there.

After being checked in, we were led to our slot in the ward. There were curtain partitions created in the ward and besides the patient bed, there was just enough space for one foldable chair / sleeper in the partitioned area. Dr. Peña and his team visited us later that day and informed us of the operation that was to be done the following day. That night, my parents called me from India on my cell phone while I was in the hospital ward. They wished us well for the important life-changing surgery that was about to happen the next day. As they spoke with me, I could not help but realize the rather loud chanting of Indian shlokas (hymns) by a number of people in my parents' house from where they were calling.

My parents explained that they had arranged for a "maha-puja" – a grand prayer to the Gods by inviting twelve priests who sang religious shlokas and mantras, sometimes individually and often times in unison. It was beautiful, heart-warning, inspiring and invigorating for me to know how intensely my parents were praying by themselves as well as the thoughtful and kind gesture they had thought of, by arranging the prayer ceremony in their house. Utilizing the miracle of technology, I was able to place my cell phone by Rajan's ear as the holy words and scriptures chanted by the Hindu priests back in India made their way through the cell phone receiver into Rajan's ear thousands of miles away in Long Island, NY.

The name of the surgery to be performed on Rajan is called "PSARP" – which stands for Posterior Sagittal Ano-rectoplasty. It is also commonly referred to as Peña's procedure – named after the great Dr. Peña who pioneered this procedure which was a radical advancement over previous surgical approaches. The PSARP offered significant advantages in terms of easier and clear access to the anatomy that needs to be corrected and minimizes any collateral damage to the surrounding nerves and urinary system organs adjacent to the site of the operation.

Two important advancements had happened in the history of colorectal surgery – and both were related to a better appreciation of the anatomy of the patient. The first was the effective use of the distal colostogram, so that the surgeon has a chance to "see" where the distal colon ends BEFORE he starts operating and does not go in blind into the surgery. Secondly, using the posterior sagittal approach has enabled surgeons to avoid nerves that used to get damaged in previously popular anterior approach methods.

Knowing that Dr. Peña was going to perform the Peña procedure gave us an enormous boost of faith and confidence we needed to think positively about the outcome of this operation. There was not a lot of prep work that needed to be done the night before the surgery except for placement of peripheral IVs in his arm. This was about the age where Rajan had somehow developed a habit of sucking the middle and ring finger of his right hand.

We figured that it was his way of calming himself. For a child who was about to undergo his third surgery in his first six months of life, letting him use whatever he liked to comfort himself as he endured all the pain that came with medical procedures and surgeries – was the least we could do for him. We requested the phlebotomist to use his left arm for IV placement, so that his right hand would stay accessible to him.

Because of the long duration of the surgery (at least 6 hours), Dr. Peña, during his rounds had advised us to go back the Ronald House while the surgery was being performed. His advice made perfect sense, since waiting in the ward seemed awkward and there really was no other designated surgical waiting area as such. Before we knew it, the time had come. They came to wheel away Rajan to the operating room and we had to re-live the moment of giving him kisses and watching him disappear on the stretcher, while handing him over to the operating team.

I held Sheri in my arms as tears flowed down our cheeks. At moments like these, the whole world becomes like an alien place, the surrounding sights and sounds blur into oblivion and a singular thought and focus of care and safety of your child becomes the center of the universe. With heavy hearts and anxious minds, we walked back to the Ronald McDonald House and entered the quiet bedroom. Letting someone operate on your child is perhaps the highest level of trust one can have in another person's ability. But regardless of the trust, leaving your child in the hands of the operating team makes you feel a kind of vulnerability and worry like no other situation in life.

I had tried to read up on a fair amount of information on this surgery and on Dr. Peña. Most of the information however, was in the form of published medical papers and while I got the gist of what the surgery was about, not having the advantage of the clinical background knowledge, made the papers difficult to fully understand. The ability to understand, absorb and interpret medical information in published papers would improve for me over time, but for now our best understanding of the surgery was that the two stomas were to stay where they were on the abdomen, while the reconstruction was to take the distal end of the colon and "pull it through" the girdle of muscles and then re-suture everything – but also create the end of the colon to now be labelled as the newly created anus. The repair or reconstruction would then need to heal over at least a couple of months after which everything would be put back together in an operation called Colostomy closure.

But for now, there were still significant challenges associated with the "pull-through procedure" (another name for the PSARP), since one of the major concerns and hence limiting factors of success, is the extent of distal colon preserved in the body to be able to extend the colon to the new site of the anus. This length in turn depends upon two factors – the intrinsic anatomy of the patient and also most importantly, where the separation of the descending colon was made to create the initial colostomy including the site where the mucous fistula is located.

Based upon medical literature, a common error caused by inexperienced surgeons is to leave to small portion of the distal colon inside the abdomen, making the PSARP surgery difficult or sometimes even impossible. Indeed there are cases, where the PSARP surgery has to be abandoned. Despite the anger that lingered inside me regarding the cosmetically unclean job" that Dr. G had performed on his colostomy surgery, I was still eternally thankful for Dr. G. having left adequate length of the distal colon for Dr. Peña to do the PSARP – as we would find out later.

CHAPTER 29: THE PSARP OPERATION

As we waited in the dark room in the RMH, Sheri and I spoke very little. We were told that we would be advised on the status through the various stages of the surgery through the landline telephone in our bedroom in the Ronald McDonald House. It was almost an hour later that the phone rang and a slightly muffled voice on the other end of the line stated "The surgery has begun. We will let you know the status of the surgery from time to time". The first milestone – start of the surgery had arrived – the journey of the surgery had begun. We waited and we waited… time seemed to pass at an excruciatingly slow pace. There was nothing we could have done or said to take our minds away from the fact that an incredibly important surgery was taking place on our six month old baby a few hundred feet away from us in the hospital's operating room.

We chose to simply endure the passage of time through silence. We wanted the room to be incredibly quiet so that nothing on earth could ever take us away from being able to hear the all-important ring of the telephone. I daydreamed and I perhaps even hallucinated that the phone was ringing and neither of us were awake to take the call because we were knocked out. Various absurd scenarios kept trying to enter and occupy my mind and I kept on driving the automatic negative thoughts out of my mind and yet they kept coming back.

I paced the room and kept changing my position every 15 to 20 minutes. Every once in a while Sheri and I would talk – and it would inevitably be about how long it has been and about why the phone has not rang yet and about what that could mean. We knew that speculations are all we had and although they had no merit, they also had no competition because of absence of any other information to replace them.

We would often then sit by each other and hold each other's hands, hoping that our clasped hands would somehow translate and transfer good luck and positive energy to influence success and a good outcome for our baby. It also seemed to bolster our mental courage and strength to endure the wait and look forward to the result. After almost another 3 hours (which seemed to last an eternity), the phone rang and startled us. I picked it up and answered it in a dry but eager voice.

A nurse spoke and the spoken words didn't match our expectations. We were expecting the phone call to indicate the end of the surgery, instead she stated that various complexities have caused the operation to be delayed, but it is still going well. I wanted to ask more details but that is all we got. As I relayed the message to Sheri, I knew that the inadequacy of the detail would get both of us worried even more. The anxiety levels in our minds rose to unprecedented levels.

There is a lot of research on the topic of stress, especially medical condition related stress. While assessing and classifying anxiety in categories such as low anxiety, state anxiety (triggered by stressful situations) and trait anxiety (innate high anxiety for seemingly minor stressful situations) can be helpful in treating patients undergoing therapies more effectively, there is not a whole lot that is applied to patient's caregivers. When you are caring for a little loved one who is sick, there is perhaps a useful property as much as a harmful property that accompanies chronic stress in caregivers. It may be hard for a researcher studying this from the outside to understand and appreciate the useful aspect of the caregiver's stress.

Caregivers, and especially parents, carry an automatic natural innate feeling of responsibility for their children. In everyday life, this does not show in a prominent way, but in sickness it gets vastly amplified. It could be the survival of progeny that becomes the supreme thought, often overriding even self-preservation. Unfortunately, chronic conditions require long term care and vigilance and letting your guard down was just not in our vocabulary – still isn't. Lower levels of stress bring about relaxation and vice versa, but come with the drawback of lower levels of vigilance. The vigilance and advocacy aspects of parents are still extremely critical aspects of caregivers attributes, but it is very hard for the brain to distinguish between the controllable and uncontrollable situations. So, by default, the brain triggers the high stress response in all stressful situations where your child's health is threatened or has potential to be harmed.

The concept of surgery is perhaps the pinnacle of this aspect as it is difficult to imagine any scenario more nerve wrecking than your child being under anesthesia, cut open and repaired. So… the agonizing wait continued for another incredibly long three hours, which was followed by a phone call that sounded like music to our ears.

CHAPTER 30: SIGH OF RELIEF

The surgery was finally over and they had begun the suturing process. We rushed to the hospital. Upon arriving, we were asked to wait in the waiting area and in a few minutes, Dr. Peña in his scrubs came to talk to us. He walked toward us with a smile and then turned his face to a neutral expression. He started off by stating that the surgery had gone well. He went on to explain that the repair surgery often takes much longer than expected because of challenges associated with the often inadequate length of the distal colon left for the surgeon to pull through.

Only experienced colorectal surgeons like Dr. Peña have perfected the art of conducting a previous surgery (colostomy) with the vision of the aspects that would facilitate the next surgery (PSARP). However, he was happy with the technical results of the surgery. We were not just happy but THRILLED to hear this news. Sheri instinctively gave a big hug to Dr. Peña. No amount of "thank you"s would do justice to expressing our gratitude for what had just happened. Maybe this was just another day in the life of a surgeon, but I couldn't help wonder if Dr. Peña realized how he had through this complex surgery created the first foundational step toward an improved prognosis and life for our son.

After the small briefing by Dr. Peña, we entered the recovery unit of the surgical ward where the overall atmosphere was quiet, except for the noises of monitors. We were led to the bed where Rajan lay – his little body covered with leads, wires, and tubes which were connected to monitors, while IV fluid and antibiotic bags hung from a pole near his bed. He had still not come out of his anesthesia and his overall status could be assessed primarily through the monitors that read and displayed his heart rate, breathing rate and oxygen levels. He was heavily bandaged in the abdomen and pelvic areas.

A small firm plastic board supported the IV line that entered his forearm by the elbow area. The board was held in place with a bandage that was wrapped around his forearm. This part of the paraphernalia was created to help maintain the IV line in proper position as it travelled for a portion parallel to his arm by being taped at multiple locations and then looped and connected with a bag supplying IV electrolytes. Sheri talked to Rajan occasionally and gently caressed his head while I just sat and watched and soaked in the situation with all of its audio visual inputs through a wide open channel that bathed my brain's entire sensory cortex.

CHAPTER 31: RECOVERY

Things progressed well and within an hour, Rajan was transferred to the general surgical ward again. It was now late evening and Rajan was awake but often dozed off because of his age (five months old) and because of the last remnant effects of anesthesia. His stats stayed stable for the most part of the time and every so often the monitor beeped – but was mostly related to a poor connection between the lead and the monitor. His IV electrolytes and post-surgical antibiotic doses continued to be delivered for the rest of the evening and they were to be removed the next day assuming his recovery continued as planned and expected. I went to the nearby LIJ cafeteria and grabbed us dinner - sandwiches which we both ate. It was now time to execute our plan – Sheri left for the Ronald McDonald house – although a bit reluctantly since she wanted to be with Rajan as much as I did.

I stayed back and had already come prepared with a pair of pajamas and toothbrush and toothpaste to stay the night with Rajan. A clipboard with instructions including those for NPO hung by Rajan's crib. He cried once in a while, but was a brave trooper through all of this. Perhaps he was still very tired because of the surgery and the medications which also included pain medications to help him cope with the variety of surgical site related pains that would start making their presence felt as soon as the anesthesia wore off. I was still very new to the experience of staying at the hospital as a caregiver. It was not like there were instructions provided for caregivers for things to be aware of or to look out for. So it was pretty much – learn as you go.

Nurses came and checked on him in the early part of the night. The frequency of their check-ins seemed to taper off as it got later into the night. We were surrounded by other patients and separated just by curtains. There were occasional conversations to be overheard, but by and large the surrounding ambience was filed with monitor beeps which appeared to be going off at random times. I am not sure what it was about the place, but something felt strange and out of place. Maybe it was the adrenalin, maybe it was heightened anxiety, whatever it was – I had an impending desire to stay alert. Since there was not much I could do about this feeling, I decided to just let it ride. The patient ward became very quiet as the night progressed.

I alternated between strolling by Rajan and keeping an eye on him, to taking a stroll just outside the ward to see the layout of the place and then back to our quarters where I would try to lay down and maybe get some sleep. But sleep seem to evade me and despite being very tired by now, I was still very AWAKE. I was not too impressed by the system in the pediatric ward as no one had come and explained any protocols to me. It almost felt like the staff was oblivious to the presence or absence of caregivers. Occasionally I sipped on my water bottle which was now empty and needed a refill. It also however meant that I had to relieve myself. I looked at the time and it was about 2:00 am. The more I thought about going to the bathroom, the more pressure I felt on my bladder.

There was no staff around our ward although I did see some occasional traffic in the corridors. I did not know where the bathrooms were, so I would have to walk around and find out. While I could have very well done that, I (for some reason) I chose not to. But I waited – thinking that I would go looking for the bathroom only after someone would come to the ward at which time I could request them to keep a watch while I went.

That proposition too seemed strange, so another option could be that I just try to hold it till morning the next day until Sheri came in – but that was at least 5 hours away. Then I noticed someone approaching our ward. It was a medical assistant. He went from bed to bed and was taking vitals.

As he approached our bed, I was a bit startled when he reached for Rajan's diaper. He had a thermometer out and was about to use the thermometer to take the rectal temperature. I was alarmed – this didn't make sense. Also, out of the instructions listed, there was also an instruction that stated "NO Rectal temperatures to be taken". It was dark and perhaps this medical assistant had not read the instructions? As he proceeded, I immediately confronted him and informed him that the instructions were clear – there was not to be any rectal temperatures to be taken on our baby – he had just come out of colorectal surgery – for crying OUT LOUD! The assistant didn't respond to me and started pointing to his clipboard – indicating to me that he was trying to do his job. He spoke almost no English and had a Russian / Eastern European accent.

I was now in front of him – blocking him from Rajan and demanded that he back off and call a nurse. Whether he understood English or not –he did understand that I was an irate dad who was not going to let him touch Rajan until the matter was clarified. The nurse on the ward heard the commotion and came to ask what the matter was. I explained to her and she totally concurred stating the obvious. But what the hell was the matter with this guy? – I demanded.

The nurse took him away to another area and a small team appeared - which may have included a translator who helped get the message across to him. When the nurse returned – I asked her what was going on and she mentioned that the hospital had hired a few immigrants and assigned jobs to them without a test of competency in spoken or written English, since the jobs were fairly straight forward and their basic medical qualification was deemed appropriate. I was not sure how true any of these statements were – but what I saw happen in front of my eyes – was that a real dangerous situation had been created. Out of ignorance or maybe out of a language barrier, one medical assistant was about to cause damage to the area that Dr. Peña and his team had worked so hard the previous day. Not only that – the repercussions of further surgical work may have very well be required due to ignorance and negligence on the part of the medical assistant.

I myself am an immigrant – I came from India to the United States and worked my way through school and my work visas and obtained a green card. I am a big believer in diversity and equal opportunity – but NEVER at the expense of poor care or substandard results. As a matter of fact – diversity or not, I expected zero tolerance for any medical errors – period. If the expected performance quality of the products I manufactured at work (fuel senders, mass air flow sensors and cruise control circuit boards was expected to be in single digit defects per million, then why shouldn't execution of healthcare be expected to not just meet but exceed automotive product quality standards? After all, you would be a lot less distressed over a faulty fuel gage than you would be with a stupid error that can damage and destroy results of a painstaking injury – right?

I stood there shaking and stunned at what had happened – mostly contemplating about what did NOT happen – but could very well have – had I not been there. Me hesitating to go the bathroom was perhaps not that silly, but rather one of many divine interventions. From my knowledge of safety and reliability at work, my brain was ready to contemplate a long series of systematic thoughts constructed in analyzing this "near miss" incident and a host of interventions to avoid and eliminate its occurrence in the future.

Adrenalin and activation of the sympathetic nervous system had peaked so high in my body that I couldn't think any more. A whole hour had passed as this event and its consequential discussions and contemplations had transpired. A few things had become clearer in my head. I quickly summoned for our ward nurse who I had complained about this incident to and simply asked her to stay at Rajan's bedside and WATCH him while I went to the bathroom. The nurse couldn't help but smile and assured me stating that she would not move an inch until I was back.

By the time I got back, I realized that my hypervigilance was gone, mostly because I thanked God knowing that Rajan was ok. My heart rate was back to normal and I felt very tired and sleepy. It was as if the parasympathetic nervous system was in control and it was demanding for me to lay down and sleep. It was as if whatever danger there was – had passed and for at least a short time, I should sleep and sleep I did.

CHAPTER 32: THINGS GOING RIGHT

I realized that it was 6:30 am and Sheri had arrived early at the hospital from the Ronald McDonald House. I was so relieved to have her back in the ward. I told her the story and watched her get furious and quickly return to feeling fortunate that Rajan was safe and that his recovery could proceed as planned and expected. Everything looked so much better and brighter on this day.

The sun was shining, and the doctors' rounds took place shortly. I brought up the issue – so they would know (which they did since the head nurse had informed them) but more importantly - focused mostly on hearing how the doctors felt his recovery was going. Dr. Peña gave Rajan's recovery a big thumbs up and prophesied that all indications pointed to a discharge on the following day.

The day progressed with Rajan being a lot more alert and active and it felt wonderful to watch him shed his leads and IV line. He returned to his regular feeding by late afternoon and with the exception of surgical site care, he looked like a healthy baby with no signs of any medical procedure, let alone a major surgery. This was the magic of not just modern science, but of how resilient babies are.

On the following day, we got discharged from the hospital as promised. We received surgical site care instructions and a date for a follow up visit in the next four days with Dr. Peña. Rajan's management had not changed, since the colostomy was still intact. The portion of the colon that had been reworked and reconstructed was still by and large undisturbed and still isolated form the rest of the alimentary canal. This was a good thing as that entire area needed time to heal.

The Ronald McDonald house often had a volunteer group come and make lunch and most times, there would be left-overs from lunch still available at dinner time.

Every once in a while, volunteers cooked dinner for the guests of the house as well. We had not had a chance to stock our basket in the refrigerator or the pantry. So, we ventured to go grocery shopping that evening. Baby Rajan was ever so eager to get in his car seat and enjoy the ride in my car. Content with his two fingers in his mouth, he relaxed in the car seat as I drove around the neighborhood in search of a supermarket. We returned with some groceries and essentials in about an hour.

On Sunday of that weekend, we were pleasantly surprised by a special brunch made by volunteers at the house. They had hearty breakfast items like eggs, bacon, hash browns, biscuits and gravy etc. But even more special was the decoration in the dining area of the house.

Everything looked bright – the table cloths were bright and each table had a bouquet of yellow lilies placed on it. On one of the walls was a banner that read "Happy Mother's day". It was indeed a very special day for all of us but especially for Sheri as she had gotten one of the most precious gifts a mother could get – a better prognosis for the life for our son.

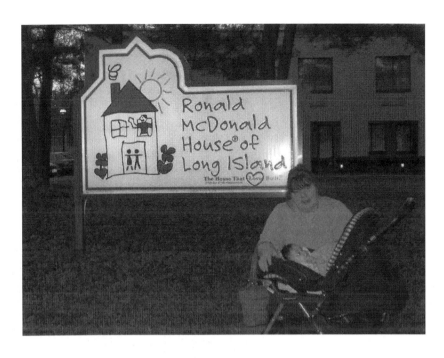

Sheri and Rajan at RMH on Mother's day

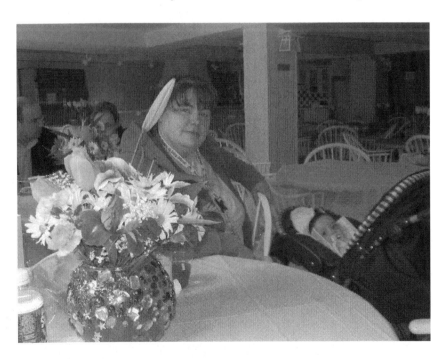

CHAPTER 33: BLISSFUL HEALING

Discharge from the hospital on the 3rd day felt sort of miraculous to us, especially in contrast to the 45 day hospital stay we had in the hospital when he was born. A week after his surgery, the day of the follow up appointment with Dr. Peña had arrived. He was pleased to see good recovery in Rajan and there were no signs of any surgical site infections. The doctor being pleased with the results made us feel even more pleased with everything since it was complimented with the general return to status quo for Rajan.

In a way, for an operation like this, functional success can only be realized after the colostomy closure operation is performed which was going to be done in a few months. Being infection free and correcting the anatomy is the major reason and objective of this operation. *The PSARP when performed in the recto-urethral prostatic fistula malformation patients (like Rajan) should result in the following anatomical and physiological improvements:*

      a. Meticulous and skillful separation of the colon from the urinary tract system (in case of the recto-urethral prostatic fistula – it would mean the disconnection of the fistula connecting the end of rectum and the ureter at about the prostate level)

      b. Successful reconstruction of the distal colon through creation of a new rectum and anus.

While a lot of emphasis is placed on part b mentioned above – mostly because the effects of part b are clear, concrete and visible, "part a" is just as important and critical. In case of Rajan, we had realized – how devastating the effects of this fistula can be. As I reflected back on the weeks following his colostomy operation in Flint six months previous, I realized that Rajan had needlessly suffered from two severe urinary

tract infections in his first six months of life because of mismanagement of prophylactic antibiotics as they were stopped prematurely. Even if the distal colon is not holding or excreting stool, as an organ
it is fully capable of harboring bacteria that belong there – which could very well make their way to the urinary tract system through the fistula no matter how small and cause BIG HAVOC thereafter.

As a dad, I was furious when I reflected on the aftermath of the medical mismanagement in the past weeks. Was this the norm, or did Rajan just happen to be in the minority proportion of patients who are unfortunate enough to experience so many complications? These were very difficult questions even for a M&M (Morbidity and Mortality) conference. While it may be hard to call something right or wrong, the reality is that medical and surgical mistakes happen a lot, and more are lost, un-identified and forgotten compared to those that make news or become the basis of law suits.

What price should patients and society pay for inexperience and ineptitude, especially if these are so hard to define in medicine currently? One incorrect medical decision or surgery, unfortunately may often result in a series of future unnecessarily exacerbated treatments or complex surgeries. As I would learn from personal experience, there is always a price to pay for mistakes and mismanagement in healthcare.

CHAPTER 34: POST-OP RECOVERY AT RMH

At the one week follow up visit, Dr. Peña also examined his stiches which were dissolvable and healing and fusing well. The highly skilled and meticulous master craftsman that Dr. Peña was, he showed off his skills by letting us examine the site and promised us that the scar left from the surgery would be very hard to detect in a few months. This can happen only when you encounter surgeons who are obsessively dedicated to their work and for whom surgery is not just a series of actions, but a work of art and joy in realizing the fruits of its outcomes through functional and cosmetic results. He also gave us a heads up about starting anal dilations in the following week.

Sheri and I were also taught the method for double diapering for Rajan, He was discharged with a catheter going into his bladder. In order to keep the surgical area clean and unexposed to urine, a hole is made in the outer diaper through which the outlet end of the catheter is passed. This ensures that the urine discharge from the catheter collects in the space between the inner and outer diaper.

Now that Rajan was doing well and traversing the path of recovery without hiccups, my attention diverted to my job and employment which had seen very little of me and my contribution lately. While I was fortunate enough to have a very understanding and compassionate boss, I also did not want to take advantage of the situation or risk losing my job.

But only after knowing that Sheri felt totally comfortable staying back for another week at the Ronald McDonald House to care of Rajan, did I make a decision to head back home. Before leaving, we spent a few days together and experienced the joys of a relatively reduced stress life and especially enjoyed the moments and memories we formed at the Ronald

McDonald house of Long Island, as we bonded with other families living there. We shared stories and always marveled at how hope and faith fueled our journey. We admonished the promise and potential of a good outcome that shone like the light at the end of the dark tunnel of illness, surgeries and treatments.

The day after our one-week follow up visit with Dr. Peña, we began researching the topic of "anal dilations". We requested use of the Ronald McDonald House office computer to look up and order a set of anal dilators. The term used is "Hegar" Dilators. They are made of stainless steel and are available from surgical specialty stores. We were given a brochure with the contact information and used the internet to order these so that they would be shipped and be available at the second week visit with Dr. Peña.

We were also advised that they do not accept insurance and that the dilators protocol was an essential part of post-surgical therapy. The thought of us as parents inserting a steel rod (dilator) through the anus of our child simply gave us chills and sounded horrible, mean and disgusting at first. All parents go through this phase, get over it and then go on to doing what is required for the betterment of their child.

CHAPTER 35: DÉJÀ VU – HOMECOMING 2

The day for me to leave back for Michigan had arrived. With bitter sweet moments of separation (sad that I had to leave Sheri and Rajan behind; yet happy that I could reunite with Roshan who was badly missing his parents). I started my journey early in the morning and was in aggressive traffic of the expressways leaving out of Long Island. Once I got out of the state of New York and into Pennsylvania, the traffic had subsided. Through the whole journey, my thoughts alternated between how Sheri and Rajan would deal with the rest of their stay in New York by themselves, to how Roshan must have been dealing with living with his grandma and aunt with no prior experience of living with them before hand, and with what work had in store for me after yet another two week absence.

This time, the sun was beating down really hard on me through the un-tinted glass of my car's windows and wind shield. About halfway through the journey, I realized that my eyelids were shutting, so I took the exit to the next rest area and parked my vehicle. I kept it running and had my car's air conditioner turned up high to counter the heat from the bright late spring sunshine. I went to the backseat, created a pillow from rolling up a few clothes, locked the car from inside and fell asleep. I was quite surprised to realize that I had slept for a whole hour in the backseat of my car.

Thanks to the versatility of the energy source of gasoline, I had effectively used the artificially created cool environment of the air conditioner in my car to enjoy a much needed nap, but I woke up stuffy – exactly what prolonged exposure to air-conditioned air does. Well – it was time to get out of the back seat – stretch, take my bathroom break at the rest area and hit the road! Several hours later, I arrived at my mother in law's house and was greeted by a hug from Roshan like never before. I could sense how much he had missed us and how glad he was for me to reunite with him.

He was only three after all. I thanked Sheri's mom and sister for all their help and left for home with Roshan.

The next week was a bit challenging – trying to get Roshan to the daycare, going to work, buying groceries, keeping the house in somewhat decent shape, making dinner etc. For now, we were in a much better place overall – Roshan and I were happy that the two of us (half the family) was at least united and Rajan was recovering well from his surgery surrounded by love and care from his wonderful mama. Even though times were tough, we felt grateful every day for every incremental progress we experienced. Rajan's appointments with the surgeon remained uneventful – which was good news. Simultaneously, information coming from the medical personnel started becoming more understandable and absorbable.

The mind needs to collaborate with the brain for "effective acknowledgement and learning" to happen. When there is excessive looming stress and worry, the simplest of things can be difficult to register and assimilate in the brain. After the large initial fog of worry and anxiety had cleared, and the promise of progress and the distant yet assuring sight of a good functional outcome started becoming more and more clear in our eyes, our resolve and confidence began to grow – slowly but surely.

Then – just like that the day had arrived when Sheri and Rajan were coming home. After purchasing a one-way ticket from La Guardia New York to Detroit, MI, Roshan and I waited with eager anticipation and a bouquet of flowers in our hands at the arrivals section of the airport on the day our family would be reunited again. A major transformation had occurred inside Rajan's body and he was half way there –

technically his rectum had been put in place and a new anus created, while the colostomy in the descending colon had yet to be reversed. In the meanwhile, it was back to our routine of managing and maintaining his colostomy. By this time, we had become experts in colostomy care. It had become a part of life and the view of the stomas when we changed bags somehow felt like any other visible part of his baby anatomy. Relieving trapped gas from his colostomy bag started to feel not terribly different than just the good old flatulence and we learned how to not be nauseated by it.

Treating Rajan's occasionally inflamed and irritated skin around the stoma started feeling not that different from a diaper rash that a child his age occasionally has. In other words, our senses went through a natural transformation of the required amount of desensitization combined with an ability to perceive a new and different, but equivalent "normal" started taking root in our brains.

CHAPTER 36: THE INSURANCE AFTERMATH

As we prepared for our upcoming challenges in the future for Rajan's continued treatment in line with his roadmap, there was another kind of transformation taking place in the treatment centers of New York and Cincinnati. Dr. Peña and his team had made their transition from Children's Hospital S in New York to Cincinnati Children's Hospital. Indeed this was a huge deal and I can only imagine how difficult this must have been for the patients and families who were accustomed to getting care at that location – to now figure out how to continue with receiving care.

For us, this was a blessing – since he was moving from being 11 hours drive to being 5 hours away (by car). In the next few months, as Rajan's protocol and condition management stabilized, a new storm raised its ugly head and began to consume us. The hospital bills started coming in... and filling our mail box. The contents of the bills were confusing, mysterious and had outrageous "out of pocket" amounts due.

Then began the phone calls – many by Sheri to the insurance companies – who directed us to the hospital billing departments and when we talked to the hospital billing, they would direct us back to the insurance company. In short – there was little communication and understanding between the two and neither was interested in minimizing the financial burden of the hundreds of thousands of $ that we now supposedly owed in the form of hospital and physician charges.

After numerous phone calls resulting in anger, frustration and confusion, it turned out that that one of the root causes of the large "out of pocket" expenses was that the hospital and its services were considered by my insurance as "out of network".

For the insurance company – this was a simple matter: "Out of network" = "Out of pocket"= "Screw the customer"! There was no attempt to communicate and understand the circumstances, or procedures that may have been required to appreciate the complexity of the situation and our rationale behind what had prompted us to seek care at this supposedly "out of network" hospital. It also turned out that there was a pre-authorization process step that was supposed to be followed before an attempt to seek care at an out of network hospital was obtained.

For any parent of family that gets news about having a child with a birth defect, which necessitates surgery within the first two days of life, followed by a month long hospital stay, two additional months of medical mismanagement of the disease resulting in multiple infections and rounds of antibiotics and then the discovery of the expertise of such treatment, trips to the location and getting through all of this challenge and trauma... when exactly should we have thought about asking our insurance company – oh, by the way, could you please enlighten us on all the paperwork we must complete before we get surgical interventions for our child? And also..."What is your opinion on whether we should seek this further treatment at the hospital with expertise in this rare condition?" and pray "Could you please approve this pre-authorization?"

My entire body fumed with rage and disgust for the ridiculously insensitive, impractical and uncooperative healthcare system we had found ourselves in. At this point of time, the hospital was interested in nothing other than recovering its money and the insurance company wanted to have nothing to do with this, since we had obviously not followed the freaking rules and procedures before doing what we did. Our struggles with the insurance and hospital billing department continued for a good six months comprising of phone calls, letters, adjusted bills, more phone calls, calls from billing debt collectors, etc. What credit card companies and banks had never done to us yet, healthcare had accomplished in a hurry – humiliating and harassing us for non-payment when there was not even clarity established in who should be paying and how much.

It was time to put our "thick skin" on and shove the responsibility back on them until we had resolution. We retaliated stating that we refuse to pay until the hospital and the insurance communicated and struck some kind of balance and covered what insurance is required to and should cover, before we figure out what our portion of the payment is. While all this financial billing chaos was in progress, we had turned our focus to the more important "next step" in Rajan's medical and surgical management per his roadmap.

Within the next 3 to 6 months, Rajan was supposed to have the colostomy closure operation – one that would reverse his colostomy and connect the two stomas back and tuck them inside neatly – where they belong. It would also be an operation that "resets" the normal functionality of the entire GI system (without any bypass) a.k.a. -in its entirety for the first time in his life! It was going to be as if his fully functional GI system would be born and where the distal colon would experience and process stool for the first time ever!

This physiologic miracle of the passage of bowels (one that few people are interested in – let alone get excited about) felt like watching the physiology of the human excretory system unravel itself in front of us in slow motion. The worry and excitement centers of my brain lit up at the same time, leaving me feeling like a confused, yet excited curious dad with an engineering mind processing biological phenomenon while being worried and anxious about what this actually meant for our son.

CHAPTER 37: BUILDING CONFIDENCE

After having met with Dr. Peña, my interest and enthusiasm about colorectal surgeries, outcomes and management had grown exponentially and the links on the first 10 pages of Google results corresponding to the search of "anorectal malformations" had been clicked on and researched to the best of my ability and understanding (which was still in its infancy at the time). The information on the internet was (and still is) quite daunting for the common person to understand, although many pediatric hospitals with colorectal centers have recently added a lot more "patient/family friendly" versions of colorectal defects management information on their websites through the form of short videos, brochures, frequently asked questions, etc.

This level of information was pretty much non-existent in 2005. So my next best bet (after downloading as many clinical research papers as I could) was to look up books on anorectal malformations and surgery and purchase them on amazon and other book selling online websites. My bookshelf now began to fill with books like Nelson Textbook of Pediatrics, Atlas of Anorectal Surgery, Anorectal Malformations in Children: Update 1988 (March of Dimes Publication) and Anorectal Malformations by Chatterjee.

Many of the books I found were old editions and much of the material had been superseded by more recent research in current day practice. I found the March of Dimes Publication to be the most relevant and useful since it was arranged in chapters which corresponded to specific malformations and its treatment standards and each chapter had different / various authors – so in a way, the book was a collection of papers / chapters written by expert authors in the field. However, none of the material was understandable mostly due to my inability to understand the terminology used in the text. So, I had to frequently refer to the Nelson Pediatric text and occasionally to select few Gray's anatomy text chapters.

On the bright side of things, our initial experience with Cincinnati Children's Hospital was good and rewarding. The hospital representatives from the colorectal center (which was just getting set up) called us to discuss logistics regarding the upcoming surgery. The date of the surgery took a while to be confirmed since apparently Dr. Peña – although he had moved to Cincinnati Children's, was not yet authorized to operate in the state of Ohio, since he had not received his state license to do so.

So, we were faced with a little dilemma – wait till Dr. Peña receives his license (which was supposed to be soon – but no specific date could be guaranteed) or proceed with another colorectal surgeon who had received his license and was a mentee of Dr. Peña and had moved from New York just like Dr. Peña had. It was really a team of colorectal surgeons and nurses that had made the move together to Cincinnati – a big blow to Children's hospital S and a big blessing to Cincinnati Children's Hospital. The alternate surgeon – who had trained under Dr. Peña and was available to do the surgery – was Dr. Marc Levitt. We just couldn't imagine anyone other than Dr. Peña doing his colostomy closure operation.

Bringing a new surgeon into the picture just did not sit well with our idea of continuity and confidence in care. So, we discussed the situation with the hospital and with Dr. Peña asking about whether waiting another month or two (within which time we were hoping that Dr. Peña receives his license) would change the outcome for Rajan in any negative way. Dr. Peña assured us that a month or two of delay in doing the colostomy closure operation would be just fine, but also informed us that his colleague Dr. Levitt would be able to do just as good of a job – in case we were interested in doing the surgery earlier.

Given the background and explanation of the options, we were very clear about our decision regarding the choice of surgeon – it was going to be - Dr. Peña who would do the surgery on our precious son – Rajan. In the meanwhile, we completed "pre-authorization" forms required by our insurance (lesson learned) and realized that history was going to repeat itself in terms of uncovered charges despite completing preauthorization forms.

So, we explored other supplemental insurances and fortunately found one offered by the state of Michigan – which would essentially cover the portions of uncovered charges from our primary insurance. The extra time we got also helped us continue to navigate the discussions and negotiations with Children's hospital S.

My family kept asking me about any finances they could help with and were ready to do whatever it takes to make sure that Rajan got the best care possible. We as parents were on the same page, but I was not yet ready to burden my parents with thousands of dollars of charges, without appropriately utilizing coverage from my existing insurance to which I was paying a mighty premium for coverage.

CHAPTER 38: BETTER PREPARATION

Then, one day there came a phone call from Cincinnati Children's Hospital informing us that Dr. Peña had finally received his much awaited Ohio license. We jumped on the opportunity to grab the first available timeslot for surgery – which happened to be on the 12th of Sep. 2005. ...And just like that- we got back into the prep mode for yet another major surgery. This means a lot of things – besides checking your insurance status. The biggest aspect of planning was associated with accommodations for our older son Roshan while we were going to be away. He was only three years old and it ached our hearts to leave him behind; yet taking him with us to the hospital would be a lot worse for him – with not much for him to do and exposing him to a schedule that we ourselves were unaware of.

As soon as I called with the confirmation of the date of surgery, my parents jumped at the opportunity to help out, especially since they had not seen Rajan since his birth. Even though they were not with us during his first few months of life, their support, blessings and love were always with us. I had called them at least every other day to keep them informed of the status of Rajan's health and recovery during the entire first month of his life.

My brother and his family who live in London (United Kingdom) were also totally engaged and equally concerned and supportive. They had also offered any help – physical, financial, logistical etc. But I had chosen to ask for this help as the last resort, since they would have to travel across the Atlantic to come and help and they had two young kids of their own to take care of. However, it was comforting for me to know that my immediate family would do whatever it took, in order to ensure that Rajan had the best possible chance to battle the odds.

Although my parents were excited to come over and fortunately had their visas procured just a year ago with a validity of 10 years, there was one problem – my mom had been unwell lately due to chronic back pain. She had sought various forms of treatments, but things had not worked out well for her. I just realized that I had not asked her about her back pain in the last couple of months, nor had she mentioned anything about it, because it seemed that 90% of our phone conversations were about Rajan and his prognosis of health.

But in the next couple of weeks, they informed me that that they were ready to book their tickets to travel across the seas and arrive a couple of months before the surgery. My mom had taken a steroid injection in her back to help with relief from the pain and their focus was now centered upon getting here and seeing us – seeing Rajan for the first time.

CHAPTER 39: HELP FROM GRANDPARENTS

I went to the Detroit airport along with Roshan to receive my parents (Rajan's grandparents). After two long flights of 8 to 10 hours each, they were happy and relieved to get past the immigration and customs checks and full of joy to see us, and so were we. The presence of my parents injected more familial support for the challenge we were about to face. As we drove from the airport to our house, I could visualize the initial "sizing shock" that my parents must have been experiencing as soon as they landed.

Everyone travelling from India to the United States experiences this phenomenon of "sizing shock" (including myself – when I am coming back to the US) which is different from culture shock, since it has to do with how we perceive ourselves relative to physical dimensions of things surrounding us. Roads, cars, expressway lanes, houses, department stores... just about everything in the US is significantly larger than what you would find elsewhere in the world. My parents had come with a very specific purpose and that had everything to do with Rajan – the entire family's singular focus at the moment.

Receiving my parents at the international arrivals lounge in Detroit, MI

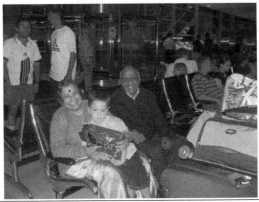

As we reached home, we noticed that Sheri had prepared a "Welcome home" sign for my parents and was right by the door as we walked in with my parents. My parents' eyes lit up and were filled with tears of joy as they held their grandson in their arms for the first time. We enjoyed the summer together, occasionally taking a dip in our pool in the backyard and going out on small trips close by so that my parents could do at least a little bit of sightseeing. There was not too much to see in the city of Flint, so we went on a small river cruise and a small train ride on the historic Huckleberry Railroad in the city. We particularly enjoyed going to the Hindu temple (every decent sized city in the US usually has one) of Flint, where we prayed together.

The next several weeks were consumed with being on the phone with the hospital to confirm details regarding the upcoming surgery, recovery from jet lag for my parents, and making logistical arrangements for my parents for their stay in our house while Sheri and I, along with Rajan were going to be at Cincinnati Children's Hospital.

We bought groceries and got my parents familiar with equipment and appliances, but they were still going to need additional help. Fortunately, our family friends (Cathy + Dave and family) were kind enough to check on them and take them to the grocery store when needed. All said and done, although we worried a little about my parents and our son being in the house by themselves, it was immensely comforting to know that they would take good care of our son Roshan while we were gone.

CHAPTER 40: HELLO CINCINNATI!

Then the day came and we set off on our car journey to Cincinnati, Ohio after the traditional spoonful of yogurt and sugar ritual that was meant to bring us good luck and a safe return. As memories of the good and bad experiences at Hospital H in Flint and Children's hospital S in Long Island, NY flashed through my mind, we looked forward to what Cincinnati Children's experience had in store for us. We certainly hoped for all the good wishes and good luck that we could garner to supplement the expertise and care he would be receiving at Cincinnati.

On the way to Cincinnati, we called to see if our request for room had been met with availability of room in the ever-so constantly occupied Ronald McDonald House – this time in Cincinnati. Unfortunately the answer was negative, so we decided to go with our plan B option as recommended by the hospital – a location called "Holmes on Eden". Our phone call to Holmes on Eden was met with a positive response for availability of one room. Holmes on Eden was a building owned by University of Cincinnati Medical Center (which is right next door to Cincinnati Children's hospital), and at the time had one floor of the building that was let to visitors seeking medical care around the area. The other floors of the building had some hospital and clinic floors and the building was only 2 to 3 minutes of walking distance from Cincinnati Children's hospital.

We arrived late in the afternoon at Holmes on Eden. The building was a bit antiquated and looked like it was in need of some renovation. The elevators were very old style and still had the "bell" sound associated with reaching the destination floor. The carpets looked worn out and the lighting was not all that great. But for some reason, none of these things bothered me much. It may have been the "singular focus" of Rajan's care in our minds or perhaps it had also to do with knowing that hotel stays (for an undetermined amount of time) were not going to be affordable or convenient (the nearest hotel was still a few miles away). So, I parked the car and we went to the registration office located on the same floor as the accommodations rooms of this hospital/hotel. The charges of the single room resembled a hotel room minus the fancy amenities. It did have a small TV, one double bed and a desk and chair.

The room felt dark even after we turned on the solitary bedside lamp. It was a bit rough on Sheri as well, when she saw the room. But she didn't complain, instead she got a box of Clorox wipes and sanitized almost all objects and things we were likely to come in physical contact with. We were also able to procure a crib from Holmes on Eden office, which we were able to somehow fit in the tight room. Just then we realized that we were starving after that long drive with no breaks other than going to the bathroom and replenishing gas in the car. We looked around and found a laminated booklet containing "take out / delivery options".

We knew nothing about Cincinnati and its restaurant options and were very hungry and tired. So, we picked this pizza delivery place called "La Rosas" and ordered one pizza and a Stromboli along with some breadsticks (which according to the specials they were running – were free). Half hour later, our cell phone rang and I went downstairs to pick up the food. The food was of typical fast food quality, but given our tired and hungry states of body and mind- it tasted like HEAVEN! Rajan was so content with his regular routine of baby food that we didn't have to worry about getting him anything from the restaurant unlike us adults who needed to.

We called home and were pleased to know that my parents and Roshan were doing well. We talked to them for a few minutes and after wishing them goodnight, were ready to go to bed.

Our physical and mental exhaustion and a carb-heavy dinner, all worked in conjunction to transport us into a much needed deep sleep – until we were both awakened by a feeling of frigid cold. We realized that the thermostat was set too low. After a few minutes of walking around the room and bumping into suitcases, table tops and bed frames, I located the thermostat and turned it up to a more comfortable setting and fell back to sleep.

CHAPTER 41: THE PROMISE OF A BETTER TOMORROW

We woke up early the following morning – in eager anticipation and filled with nervous and anxious energy of going to the hospital and getting Rajan admitted. After quick showers, we stepped out into the hallway to see what kind of breakfast was offered by this hospital/hotel. They had a self-serve continental breakfast of cereal, boiled eggs, bread, orange juice, muffins, bananas and apples and COFFEE! Again – none of it was arranged in any fancy manner – but was available for us right there. We were very appreciative of this continental breakfast and in another hour, we headed out walking from Holmes on Eden to the hospital with Rajan in his stroller. The weather was still quite a bit warmer in Cincinnati compared to Michigan.

As we entered the hospital, we were immediately struck by how enormous it was (our reference point until then were the two pediatric units of adult hospitals). We quickly learned from the signs posted in the hospital, that it was ranked "#3" in the nation based upon US News and World Report rankings of pediatric hospitals. We entered a long busy hallway in the "D building" and saw multiple signs. The hallways were called concourses and they fit the description – based upon its comparison with airports. As we walked all the way across the hallway passing clinicians, patients and family members, we soaked it all in.

This was Rajan's new place of care and it was important for us to become familiar with it. We walked all the way past buildings C, and B before we arrived in building A (all of these buildings were seamlessly connected and could very well have been just one big building in a C shape with separations simply by walls, stairwells, elevators and signs. We looked for the sign for "Admissions" and there it was – in one corner of the hospital. It was also the location for lab work. Once we announced our arrival, we were asked to wait in the waiting area. About 10 minutes later, a nurse arrived.

The nurse walked us through the admissions procedure and had us complete a few consent forms. There would be a lot more procedures of admissions to follow, but for now, we had completed enough paperwork that we could make our way to the designated hospital room located in the south wing of the fourth floor of the A building (A4-S).

We followed the nurse as we went through hallways, elevators, more hallways and into the unit of A4S. The unit looked fairly busy and was humming with occasional equipment alarm beeps and personnel walking back and forth between rooms. The first things that struck me, as I walked into the room, was the presence of its own bathroom and its own door. The room was spacious and a crib suitable for babies was placed in the room which itself appeared well equipped with every possible medical contraption that could be needed within an arm's length away.

This was actually the standard hospital room in a typical large pediatric hospital – but seemed like a 5 star hotel to us when we compared it with our previous experience. This hospital must be endowed with some incredible funding sources – I thought to myself as I contemplated the variation in outcomes in relationship to the extent of care and facilities patients received.

If the variation that one family with one condition (aka Rajan and us – his mom and dad) had seen with our own eyes, how much more variation was out there in this advanced and wealthy nation of United States and how much variation was there across hospitals in the whole wide world? My train of thought was interrupted, as an intake nurse introduced herself and greeted us. She handed us a folder with papers about the admission and about the hospital as well its features and general information about what to expect during the hospital stay. She then began to go through an intake questionnaire which spanned through a detailed medical history from his birth through the present moment.

It had been only nine months of his life, but he had accumulated a large enough medical history that most people would not experience in a lifetime. I had become somewhat of an encyclopedia of his medical history and gained the skill of being able to recite it without having to look up his records. The names and doses of his antibiotics that worked and didn't work were all on the tip of my tongue. As I listed his current status, my mind drifted to his journey with antibiotics. One encouraging aspect of progress was the stopping of his prophylactic antibiotic after his PSARP operation in June of that year. This made complete sense as the source of his earlier infections (UTIs) was the fistula – which Dr. Peña had eliminated through the surgery.

Day before surgery at Cincinnati Children's Hospital

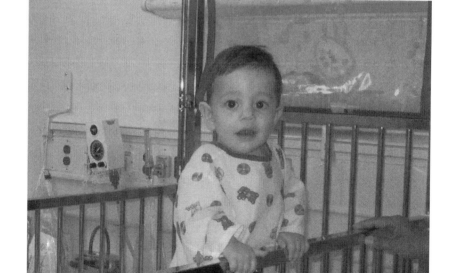

CHAPTER 42: CLOSURES

The next surgery for Rajan was supposed to be the Colostomy closure. There was not a lot of prep required for this surgery other than being NPO (no food or drink) from the night before the surgery. Surgery was going to be the next day and the time for putting in the IVs had come. The poking and prodding to find his vein always made us shudder, so this first attempt to find the vein and connect the IV felt like a big relief to us. We asked for the IV to be placed in his left arm, in order for him to be able to continue his habit of sucking his middle two fingers of his right hand.

The stage was set and Dr. Peña came and talked to us on the day before the surgery and asked us if we had any questions. His presence and confidence inspired us and made us even more hopeful of a desirable outcome form the surgery. Consent forms for surgery were signed on the day before the surgery, when a surgical resident stopped by and went over the contents of the papers. Nothing was rushed and they were all very respectful and patient with us when we did have questions. Everything appeared to be well-organized in this hospital. I stayed in the hospital room that night and as always Sheri came in early in the morning on the following day, well in time before the transporter came to get Rajan.

Day 1:
This is when it hit us – the time had come where we would have to let him go out of our sights – to undergo his transformation. But letting him go out of our sights was always so hard – no matter what the reason was. At this time, we were waiting in a small room by the operating room and the anesthesiologist came by and introduced herself. She went over some technical details and had us sign additional consent forms related to anesthesia. At this point of time, we

had no logical comprehension of what we were signing – all we looked for were signs of trust and confidence in what surrounded us and whom we talked to. If we found those two things, we went ahead. If things felt wrong, we paused and asked more clarifying questions. Our intuition had given us the "all clear" and so, we were trusting of everything that was happening. This feeling was very different than the one I had in Children's Hospital S. Rajan was still asleep as he was wheeled on the gurney from the small waiting room to the operating room. It was time to say good bye for a while. We gave him lots of kisses and wished him all the luck in the world. Our stomachs were sick with worry and our brains were mush with emotions as we watched our son being wheeled away into the operating room. We watched as the doors of the OR shut in front of us.

Then it was just the two of us –holding each other's hands as we kept staring at the closed doors of the O.R. We were then advised to go the surgical waiting area – a place specifically designed for families of patients to wait as their loved one was being operated on. The room was a large hall with lots of seats, tables, benches and sofas as well as TVs. There were two large monitors with patient numbers and the current status of the operation displayed.

Each family was given their patient's ID number so that they can track progress on the display monitor, without giving away personal information. We were also given a pager which was supposed to light up, whenever there were updates from Rajan's surgery for us while he was in the O.R. The pager, we were told would work throughout the hospital campus, so that we would be informed even if we had stepped away from the waiting room and gone to – for example the cafeteria. But we chose to go nowhere. There was a coffee machine and a vending machine with snacks. We got ourselves some coffee and then just sat there looking blankly at whatever was playing on the nearest TV. We were surrounded by families of patients who were all in the same boat – waiting to hear the outcome of surgery for their loved ones. Time always seems to crawl in situations like these and you want to just be able to jump ahead in time. But all things must happen the way they are meant to and even though the wait feels like torture, it is in some ways paying tribute to the difficult and important work going on a hundred feet away in the operating room.

Seeing other families is sometimes comforting, but in times like these, it is almost impossible to have conversations with anyone – small talk or any other talk feels like a distraction and the mind simply wants to keep thinking about what's going on in the Operating Room. We periodically checked on the status of the operation on the display board – which was the equivalent of the brief update phone calls we had received from the operating room during the last surgery in New York.

The wait was over when the pager came to life and buzzed and lit up. This was our cue to go to the front desk area of the hall and the representative collected the pager from us and informed us that they would call out our names in just a few minutes when Dr. Peña would arrive and brief us on the outcome of the surgery and about how Rajan was doing. Every second of the last part of this wait felt like being on pins and needles awaiting the result of a very important test of your life! It may have been less than two minutes, when we heard our name being called and we hurried to a small cubby-like room where Dr. Peña had just arrived.

Dr.Peña was still in his scrubs and had come straight from the O.R. He greeted us with a smile but quickly became serious and spoke in a very professional and precise language. He was kind enough to explain terminology when we struggled to understand certain words – but the take home message was clear – his closure surgery had gone very well and Dr. Peña was particularly proud of the minimal S shaped suturing he had done, the scar of which he reassured us, should be barely visible in a few months. Most importantly, he told us that the "functional" outcome of the surgery should be evident in two days. We both hugged Dr. Peña and thanked him multiple times for all he had done for Rajan thus far.

Day after surgery

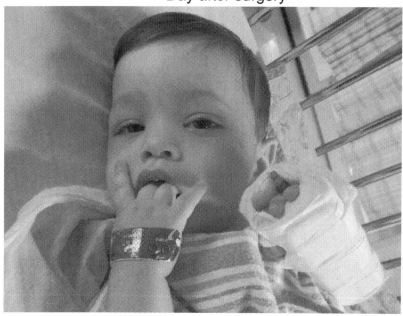

CHAPTER 43: THE BEAUTIFUL NEWS OF A SUCCESSFUL SURGERY

We were now super-anxious to see our baby. As Dr. Peña left, a medical assistant took us to the post-op recovery room. The room was only partially lit and was essentially a large hall with curtain separators. It was after all a temporary place for post-operative recovery, close to the operating room where patients were monitored for about an hour or two or until the time that they were stable and safe enough to continue the rest of their recovery in the hospital room. Rajan was yet again connected to several IVs and he lay there still, his eyes closed and his leads monitoring his vital stats. The nurse monitoring him expressed "doing great" relative to his recovery status.

We were delighted to just see him. We took turns lightly touching and holding his left hand that was free of all IVs and other paraphernalia. An oxygen mask lay next to his head facing his mouth, so he could breathe in air that was slightly richer in oxygen content. He did not need to be connected to oxygen, since he was doing well with breathing on his own and his O2 stats looked good. For the next several minutes we just sat there and watched him as he jerked randomly every few minutes as the anesthesia was slowly wearing off.

After what seemed to be about 45 minutes to an hour, they were ready to transport Rajan to his hospital room. We returned to the hospital room we had come from earlier that morning. It was early evening at this point of time and our biggest satisfaction came from him being safely situated in his crib. IV drips continued to hydrate and nourish him as he opened his eyes occasionally but generally was sleepy enough to keep drifting back to sleep after brief bouts of wakefulness. Sheri and I finally took turns to go to the cafeteria and get something to eat.

The cafeteria (although open 24 hours a day) is at its worst between meal hours. So, if you go there after lunch hours and before dinner hours started, most stalls would be closed and nothing they offer at such times is fresh, and your choices are limited. I don't remember what I got, nor was it important – just needed to get something into our stomachs that had been empty all day except for the coffee and the single vending machine snack we had in the surgical waiting hall area.

While Rajan was still recovering in the hospital room, we received a phone call informing us that a room in the Ronald McDonald house had become available. So, I went over to Holmes on Eden, checked out, and brought our supplies and personal items to the RMH (Ronald McDonald House). Later that evening, Sheri and I returned to the RMH. We registered at the RMH and were given a brief tour. After having lived in the NY Long Island Ronald McDonald house, we had become familiar with the workings of the RMH, but were still appreciative of the small tour of the Cincinnati RMH that one of the volunteers gave us.

While RMHs across the world are similar in purpose, they tend to be different in structure. After getting our lanyards and keys, we were back at the hospital. Rajan's recovery continued to go well and although our confidence with the services provided was high, there was still no way we were going to leave Rajan unattended – especially through the night. As per our protocol, I stayed the night in the room with Rajan and Sheri went to the Ronal McDonald house. The neighborhood around the hospital was not very safe and it was not recommended for ladies to walk by themselves at night outside the hospital, so one of the hospital security personnel offered to escort her on the short walk to the RMH.

There was fortunately a land line telephone in the RMH rooms. Sheri called me after she arrived in the RMH room and

I assured her that Rajan was continuing to do great and was now staying awake for longer periods of time before he kept drifting back to sleep. This was normal, since in addition to the remnant effects of the anesthesia, the pain medications also induced sleep. Sheri and I were both physically and mentally exhausted. I made a phone call to home in Michigan (where my parents eagerly awaited the news) and informed them that all was going well. My parents in turn called my brother in London to keep him informed of the progress.

I opened my sofa sleeper and laid down the sheet cover provided by the hospital and laid down. The realization of the completion of a successful surgery and closure to one critical episode of care created a calm inside my body that led me to finally relax for a little while. Soon, I drifted into deep sleep.

CHAPTER 44: CHANGING THE OUTCOME TOGETHER

My deep sleep however was only short-lived. I woke up in the middle of the night. It was dark and quiet with some light seeping in from the hallway along with the occasional beeps of the monitor and the rhythmic turning of the IV pump. Some people find the noise of monitors and IV pumps annoying and disturbing enough that they are unable to sleep. However, I found the rhythmic noises to be just fine. I did not enjoy long deep sleep, nor did I want to – after all I was in the hospital as a dad wearing the hat of a caregiver. I rested but did not fall back into deep sleep. In fact, every time the alarms went off, I was glad to be woken up, asked for the nurse if she did not show up in time, and was relieved that most alarms were false positives (as in all OK, but lead malfunctions resulting in a false alarm).

I had worked for years in the automotive industry where reducing false failures while never missing true positives were challenging projects to take on. But, here in the hospital, I was inclined for being totally OK with a slightly elevated false positive rate if it came with the advantage of an absolute zero rate of missing a true positive alarm. After checking on him, and looking around the room, I felt safe enough to return to my light sleep mode until early morning arrived. Sheri was here very early as she couldn't wait to come and see us.

Day 2: As the day after surgery progressed, Rajan's energy and alertness increased by the hour. Dr. Peña had stopped by during morning rounds with the entire rounding team and asked us how we thought he was doing. I reported stating that he had an uneventful night and smiled (as I put the bad memory of the rectal temperature attempt fiasco at Children's Hospital S from a few months ago behind me). Dr. Peña was happy with the results of the surgery and wanted him to be weaned off the IV lines by midafternoon and encouraged us to start oral feeding later during the day.

We were delighted to hear this news. As promised and expected, the IV lines came out and Sheri began to feed him with liquids and soft food before moving to his regular food as advised. Rajan did great and responded very well to his food intake. He was even up and about in his crib showing vibrant signs of a good recovery.

Day 3: The next day came about and we were now anxiously awaiting the "functional" outcome of the surgery.... The bowel sounds were good and strong and it was only a question of time before we knew if all this was actually going to work. Late in the afternoon that day, we were able to "smell" success! Yes – he had pooped in his diaper! For the first time in his life in the way we are supposed to! Never before would we have in our wildest dreams thought of being in a situation where we would be so excited about our baby pooping!

We wouldn't expect others to understand – but parents of children with an anorectal malformation will know exactly what I am talking about. It is one of the biggest milestones in the roadmap of the child with an anorectal malformation. It is the beginning of the manifestation of all things possible!

CHAPTER 45: EXPERIENCING "NORMAL"

After the successful demonstration of the "functional" outcome of the colostomy closure operation, and with continued post-surgical progress without any signs of complications, Dr. Peña was delighted to agree to discharge after another day of observation. This would be yet another successful beginning of the realization of the potential for bowel control (fecal continence) for his newest patient – and our precious son – Rajan.

- 09/11/15; Colostomy closure operation date
- 09/12/15; Post op recovery and IV removal and oral feeding
- 09/13/15; First successful functional outcome (poop)
- 09/14/15 and 09/15/15: Observation days
- 09/16/15: Successful discharge and enjoying life at the RMH:
- 09/17/15: We had a joyful day of celebration at the RMH that day; celebration of a successful surgery and a brilliant recovery. During the observation days, we started him on a daily dose of one to two drops of a baby laxative "Little Tummies" and determined two drops to be the right amount for him. We were to continue this regimen WITHOUT FAIL until he was going to be ready for potty-training, which in his case would be following a week long program of bowel management that would be done during his toddler years. But this was at least two years out. For now, he could be just like a regular baby with the addition of the daily 2 drops of Little Tummies every night. We were strongly advised to make sure that he does NOT go without a bowel movement for even a single day moving forward. We didn't quite understand the significance of this until I read about the effects of the

surgery. Even with the most skillfully executed surgery, it turns out that anorectal surgery such as PSARP and colostomy closure, inevitably induce a state of idiopathic (unknown precise cause) constipation in patients. So, the stool travels to the newly reconnected colon and rectum, but there is just not enough peristaltic movement and the associated stimulation in coordination with sphincter muscle brief relaxation (the mechanics of a bowel movement) to happen in a natural manner as it does in healthy people without this malformation.

So, a form of stimulation such as this mild laxative for now, was going to do the job. However, moving forward, this was going to be a much more complicated task – which we would deal with when he would be three years old.

CHAPTER 46: SMOOTH RECOVERY

We spent a few more days at RMH for his follow up appointments with Dr. Peña post-surgery. This time (with the travel time being a mere 4.5 hours) I decided to go back to Michigan and bring the rest of the family to come to see Cincinnati and then all of us head back home together. So, I did just that. I came back to Cincinnati with my parents and Roshan so we could see some places in Cincinnati (we went to the zoo and aquarium and while my parents and Roshan along with me stayed at the hotel for two nights, Rajan and Sheri continued their stay at the RMH.

The last post-op follow up visit with Dr. Peña went very well. We then headed back to Michigan in our Honda Pilot (thank goodness for a vehicle with 3 row seating). When we arrived, Sheri and Rajan were pleasantly surprised by the chalk art display of "Welcome Rajan" pre-done by my mom before we had left for our Cincinnati trip and a "Welcome Sheri and Rajan" paper posted on the garage door. The blissful feeling of being home after enduring the hardships of hospital stays and surgeries felt like a soothing relief over our battle wounds.

Every surgery left a physical scar on his body and a mental scar in our minds as we weathered the challenges with all the courage we could gather. Technically, this could have been the end of the roadmap for surgeries and the beginning of the medical management roadmap, but time would tell if the road we were on – still needed us to be on it. For now, we were happy to live in the moment and rejoice the "closest to normalcy" experience we had enjoyed since his birth. It had taken us a whole 11 months to get there.

As I looked around I saw Sheri holding Rajan in her arms back at home sitting comfortably in her favorite rocking chair, I thought to myself – how blessed and fortunate I was to have this moment of success, happiness, belonging, love and bliss – all rolled into one. And despite the difficulties and the troubles, I felt grateful for being in a country where the best pediatric colorectal surgeon in the world worked, and having the opportunity for him to give our son the best shot at having a life as close to normal as possible.

Dr. Peña holding Rajan:

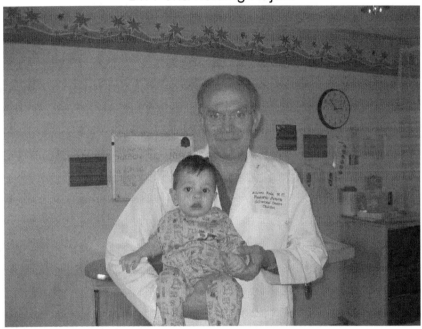

CHAPTER 47: ALL'S WELL THAT ENDS WELL

We enjoyed the company of my parents for another couple of months and they thoroughly loved their time with us and relished being in the company of their grandchildren and of our family being together. Sheri and I could not have wished for anything different or better. Everything happens for a reason. If we were meant to battle the difficulties of bringing up a child who was unfortunate enough to have a birth defect with an unknown cause, then by God – we were going to fight that battle with all the might, courage and knowledge we can and hope to come out with the best possible kind of success we can envision, that science can deliver and that hope and prayer can sustain. September was upon us now and my parents were getting ready to return to India. As we said goodbye, our hearts were filled with great love and appreciation for both of them.

We had returned to our routines by the beginning of the Fall season. The months of November and December brought plenty of snow to our city and state and the festive season was in the air. We decorated the Christmas tree with great gusto to make up for the previous year's December that was spent in its entirety in the hospital. But that was behind us. We had so much to celebrate, including Rajan's first Birthday in the first week of December. We invited friends and family to come to his 1st. Birthday celebration and for just a moment I reflected back on my mixed emotions exactly a year ago.

We had come a long way in Rajan's first year of life. It had taught us many lessons, the biggest of which were: having a positive outlook, challenging the status quo, seeking answers to difficult problems, finding expertise to solve problems, relying on family and friends, and staying united as a family. We learned that love, courage, hope and resilience are the key ingredients to overcome barriers that life throws at us. The 5000th. baby had not just survived, he had thrived and taught us all to aim and work with all we have toward nothing but the best outcome. In the upcoming years, there would be many more medical, psychosocial and financial problems to solve...but every once in a while, little miracles happen and give you strength to carry on. On Christmas-eve, we got a phone call from Children's Hospital S rom New York Long Island. The anesthesia department representative was on the other end of the line. She told us, that after review of the complicated case, the hospital had decided to waive off the $11,000 hospital Anesthesia bill that we owed. Although it was by no means the resolution to all financial issues, it was the little ray of encouraging light that encouraged us by saying "Keep going, you are doing all the right things- Merry Christmas and Happy New Year!"

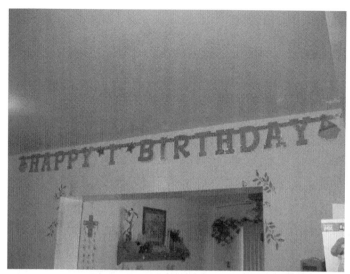

Rajan's first birthday celebration

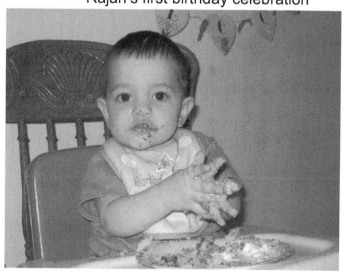

EPILOGUE

There were many bumps in the road, as we traversed our journey through the toddler and early teen years for Rajan. However with every problem, barrier and near miss incident, we rejoiced in the experience of triumph over adversity. Our list of lessons learned kept growing over time. With every physical and mental scar, our strength was tested and our resilience bolstered. Surgical management reduced over time and medical management waxed and waned.

The chronic nature of the disease created physical and psychological stress, which in turn manifested in pain. Appreciating psychologic pain became just as important as physical pain, and overcoming it taught us other lessons in chronic disease management that we were unaware of. In other words, we kept on going... taking success and setbacks in our stride and continuously pursuing a good outcome out of all of this for Rajan.

At the time of writing this book, Rajan has grown to be a strong, healthy, athletic, and academically proficient kid, who is now 15 years old. Much like his other friends, he loves to have fun, play sports (running cross country and track and basketball are Rajan's favorite sports), go on vacations with family, enjoy sleepovers at friends, and just goof around. With perseverance and practice on his own accord as well as ours as parents and family, he can now independently do all things a typical 15 year old does.

We have doctors' follow up visits with a couple of specialties in Cincinnati Children's Hospital every six months. As long as his test results continue to show a "clean bill of health", his chronic condition appears to be only in the rear view mirror. But history has taught us to be vigilant, as there is no perfect roadmap carved out for anorectal malformation patients and every patient's individual journey is different.

As I think of Rajan's first year of life and the past decade and a half, I visualize it as a collective journey of him and us as a family. Our extended family of course includes his clinicians who have played such an important role in his life and influenced his outcomes to a great extent. This young man has grown, and blossomed based upon his own resilience, will power and drive to thrive and succeed along with a little help from the loving village comprising of his family, friends, and his clinicians. No one knows the future and what impact Rajan's challenging medical issues from his childhood may have on his future, but as they say "The only way to live life is cherishing it one day at a time".

We hope this book provides some knowledge, guidance and most importantly reassurance and hope to families dealing with medical challenges for their child. Our actions and our attitude are just as important and impactful as genetic and disease-specific predisposition are, when it comes to outcomes for our precious children. May the story of the 5000th baby, and many other similar stories of children and their families overcoming adversity be the shining light that inspires us to traverse our own tunnels of life.

Difficult roads often lead to beautiful destinations.

AUTHOR'S REFLECTIONS

Psychology:

When faced with an unexpected crisis, there are two channels of thought processes related to the desire to understand and assign cause. One focusses on singular blame (fast, spontaneous assignable cause thinking) and the other utilizes a rational open minded scientific approach (slow, thoughtful and reasoning based thinking). Blame (especially self-blame) in cases of birth defects has, for many reasons been the predominant school of thought, thereby denying the rational school of thought an opportunity to influence behavior and decisions.

Birthing centers, and pediatric hospitals should be enabled with providing resources in the form of behavioral psychologists who can help provide a balanced form of thinking for parents that are exposed to such trauma, as realizing that their child has been born with a birth defect. Such a resource can lend an empathetic ear to the parents, as well as provide information in the form of guidance and resources in the right balance of quantity and timing, so that parents make the most informed decisions regarding their child's course of care.

There is a dire need for such patient/family advocates for parents and families of children born with birth defects requiring chronic disease management. Shifting the mindset from obsessing over cause to seeking effective solutions seems obvious, but is much easier said than done, when faced with crises like these.

Inequity of access and variation in exposure to evidence based science:

In the field of public health, it is often said that your zip code is a determinant of your health and outcomes. Proximity to children's hospitals and the extent of access to expertise in hospitals to medical and surgical care – especially for rare conditions continues to be the Achilles heel of healthcare quality and reliability. Often times, the lack of knowledge and access to expertise required to address time-sensitive care results in poor quality of care and thereby widens the gap in outcomes by region. Protocols and best practice standards usually exist, but are not always available, known or deployed in hospitals far away from advanced academic centers of excellence.

Whether it is management of medications (like antibiotics), or the timing of surgeries, or the prevention of avoidable surgical complications – widespread dissemination of best practices across the country and the globe can make a difference in the lives and outcomes of such children. We need a focused effort on addressing the inequities of care and outcomes by geography.

Story telling from the patient and family's perspective:

There are countless stories of successes and disasters lived and experienced by patients and families that are mostly untold, and therefore forgotten and ignored with regard to the potential they have, to transform care and outcomes for the better. Combining the knowledge of what happens outside the hospital with what happens within, will advance the science of healthcare to a new frontier. We need to create a culture of openly sharing barriers and challenges to care as experienced by patients and families as seen through "their eyes" in order to better understand, appreciate and then improve care and outcomes in a holistic manner.

APPENDIX

A. Recommended initial reading for parents of a new born child with anorectal malformation
B. First year roadmap for anorectal malformation patient
C. Ronald McDonald Houses
D. Pullthru Network
E. Stoma care
F. Helpful Do's and Don'ts for parents and families of children with anorectal malformations

A.
RECEOMMENDED INITIAL READING FOR PARENTS OF A NEW BORN CHILD WITH ANORECTAL MALFORMATION

Dear proud Parents,

First of all, congratulations on the birth of your baby! The beginning of new life is truly a reason for celebration.

FIRST THOUGHTS:

You are however, most likely experiencing two emotions at the opposite ends of the spectrum simultaneously (joy and shock) because you have just received the unexpected news of your child being born with an anorectal malformation. Understandably, the emotions are overpowering the joy and you are probably very concerned about your baby. I can relate to this experience because I happen to be a parent who experienced such intense emotions in 2004 upon the birth of our second son. I would like to share some of my own knowledge regarding this accompanied with verification of the same by medical experts in this aspect of birth defects. I hope that reading this article will educate you about this unexpected circumstance and provide you with important information to help you and the medical practitioners in your area make appropriate decisions.

Much like we experience a wide variety of emotions, anorectal malformations also happen to be of various kinds in terms of their characteristics and are often said to be on a spectrum. Anorectal malformations are birth defects where the anus and rectum (the lower end of the digestive tract) do not develop properly. The following table is based upon the modern classification of anorectal malformations.

Anorectal malformations classification [1]

Males	Females
1. Perineal fistula	1. Perineal fistula
2. Rectourethal fistula:	2. Vestibular fistula
a. Bulbar fistula	3. Persistent cloaca:
b. Prostatic fistula	*a. <=3cm common channel*
3. Rectobladder neck fistula	*b. >=3cm common channel*
4. Imperforate anus without fistula	4. Imperforate anus without fistula
5. Complex defects	5. Complex defects

UNDERSTANDING THE DEFECT:

The first and most important step is to determine the type of malformation that your child has. While disappointment may feel imminent, discouragement need not be. It is also important to acknowledge that all anorectal malformations affect bowel function. Based upon the type and severity of the defect, the prognosis of the defect can result in varying degrees of constipation or incontinence (the two extremes of the spectrum of bowel function). The prognosis is affected primarily by three factors:

a) Type of anorectal malformation

b) Surgical competence and successful execution

c) Associated anomalies (mostly sacral and spinal)

Unfortunately, improper understanding of the defect and subsequent improper treatment can lead to serious and sometimes irreparable damage that could have otherwise been avoided. Hence it is very important to understand the specific type of defect using the proper terminology as soon as possible. In some previously published literature, you may find information on classification of anorectal malformations in the categories of "high" or "low" based upon the location of the distal end of the rectum. Use of this terminology provides little or no insight into prognosis or treatment options. Hence it suggested that use of such generic terminology be avoided. Given the rare occurrence of these types of birth defects and the wide variance in the level of medical knowledge regarding these conditions, it is very important that you insist on asking for the appropriate level of expertise in getting an accurate diagnosis of the specific type of malformation. Sometimes, this may require you to obtain services from the nearest pediatric colorectal center if available and applicable.

OTHER ASSOCIATED CONCERNS:

Associated with anorectal malformations, is often the mention of the term **VATER** or **VACTERL**. The letters of this acronyms stand for defects associated with **V**ertebral, **A**nal, **C**ardiac, **T**racheo**E**sophageal, **R**enal and **L**imb. While the associated defects can sometimes be diagnosed concurrently in babies born with anorectal malformations, its generic use and reference as a diagnosis is often misleading and confusing. It is also important to realize that many babies born with anorectal malformation could have minor anomalies associated with the organs from the term but could be in the category of discrepancies that do not need interventions and will go away with time. In the interest of better understanding and clarity in communication, it is suggested that the generic reference to VATER or VACTERL be avoided.

On the other hand, unfortunately, most babies (50 to 60%) born with anorectal malformations do have one or more abnormalities that affect other systems. While the determination of the specific type of malformation is taking place, it is equally important to have the appropriate tests (most tests are done within 24 hours of life) done to determine if there are any other associated abnormalities. The probability and type of other abnormalities varies based upon the type of anorectal malformation.

The following are the most commonly occurring types of anomalies associated with babies born with anorectal malformations:

- **Cardiac anomalies:**

While these types of associated anomalies are present in almost one third of patients, only about 10% of them need any treatment. Majority of the defects are not concerns and will go away without treatment.

- **Gastrointestinal anomalies:**

There are many different types of gastro-intestinal associated anomalies and trachea-esophageal anomalies are the most common amongst them.

- **Spinal, sacral and vertebral anomalies:**

While there is again a wide variety of these types of associated anomalies, the most frequent spinal problem is *tethered cord*. A tethered spinal cord is a condition where there is restricted movement of the spinal cord, which lies within the spine, surrounded by the vertebrae.

Sacral anomalies have a strong correlation with the eventual functional outcome. One of the important ways by which the sacral anatomy is quantified is through a term called "sacral ratio". *Be sure to ask the doctors about the actual value of this ratio. Higher ratios (greater than 0.7) are indicative of more chances of success with bowel control.*

- **Genitourinary anomalies:**

The three commonly occurring urologic defects are vesicoureteric reflux, renal agenesis and dysplasia. Girls born with anorectal malformations are also susceptible to having other associated gynecologic anomalies. It is important to have knowledge of these anomalies in the new born period.

SUMMARY:

From the point of view of being a parent who has received such news, it is quite likely that you are thinking about questions such as "How did such a thing happen?" or "Why was it not detected before the birth of my child?" or "What should we do now in order to provide the best possible care and treatment for my child?" The answers to the first two questions are not yet fully known in the current state of medical science and literature. So, although they are very natural questions in your mind, it is in the best interest of your child and your family to focus on the third question. Doing this will maximize your chances of doing the right thing for your child and have a strong impact on his/her future.

So, in summary:

1. Avoid the use of terms such as "high" or "low" to describe the type of defect. Ask for an accurate diagnosis of the specific type of anorectal malformation per the new classification chart as you have seen in this article. Try to get the best expertise that you have available or can get in order to do this effectively.

2. Avoid the use of the generic term of VATER or VACTERL. Instead, make sure that your baby is examined for associated anomalies (preferably within the first 24 hours of life) with appropriate tests (such as ultrasounds of kidneys and spine, x rays of abdomen and sacrum, and cardiac echo).

3. Obtain information about immediate (short term) and long term overviews and try to get an expert opinion from a nearby colorectal center (that specializes in treatment of such conditions) as early as possible.

When my son was born with an anorectal malformation, he did not receive optimal care. I was told that my son had a long and bumpy road ahead of him but not many specifics. Over time, we as his parents have become a lot more familiar with the condition and with its management and treatment options available to us. Through a series of "colorectal pathways", I would like to present to you all diagrammatic representations of "what to expect" in the form of treatment pathways that will enable you to be more educated and more prepared to travel this journey with the hopes of good outcomes.

Thanks and regards,

Technical supervision provided by:

Alberto Peña, MD and Emilio Fernandez, MD

Written by:

Devesh Dahale   (Parent of a child born with prostatic fistula)

B.
FIRST YEAR ROADMAP FOR ANORECTAL MALFORMATION PATIENT

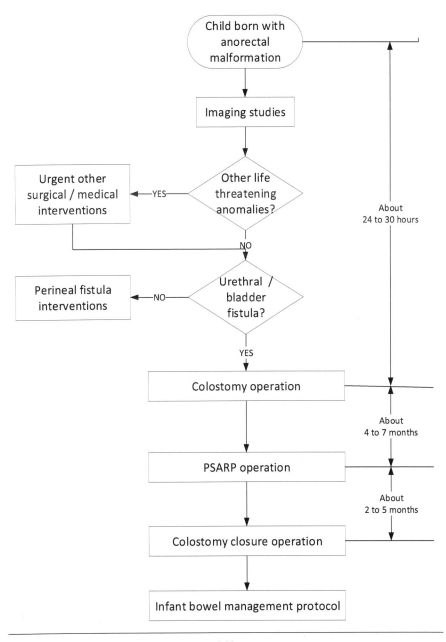

C.
Ronald McDonald Houses

For patients and families:

- If you are traveling to the children's hospital for anything more than 50 miles for your child's treatment, consider Ronald McDonald House for your lodging needs.

- Do contact the Ronald McDonald House well in advance and let them know your anticipated travel and arrival dates, as well as your child's treatment or hospital stay dates. While the House will not be able to reserve a room for you, they will add you to the wait list and contact you as soon as a room becomes available upon your arrival.

- For your child's short term or long term medical needs, staying at Ronald McDonald House provides you with the comfort of a home and proximity to the children's hospital you are seeking care at.

- Always have an alternate lodging option available until room becomes available at the Ronald McDonald House.

- The House provides you with opportunities to interact with families who are in similar situations. This can often be therapeutic in itself.

- The House will work with you to make lodging as affordable to you as possible so you can focus your energy on caring for your child rather than worrying about finances and logistics related to lodging.

For all:

Interested in donating to or volunteering for Ronald McDonald House?

Ronald McDonald Houses are funded and sustained by grants and donations from corporations, organizations and generous donors. To find out more, visit:
www.rmhc.org

To find a Ronald McDonald House near you, visit:
https://www.rmhc.org/chapter-search

D.
Pullthru Network

This not for profit organization is another resource for patient and families of anorectal malformations. Their mission statement as noted on their website is as follows:

Pull-thru Network, Inc. is a volunteer-based non-profit organization dedicated to providing information, education, support and advocacy for families, children, teens and adults who are living with the challenges of congenital anorectal, colorectal, and/or urogenital disorders and any of the associated diagnoses.

www.pullthrunetwork.org

E.
Stoma Care

Stoma care can initially feel daunting, but knowledge about your options, doing some research to find best affordable alternatives and with some practice, you can master the science and art of stoma care.

1) DO: Keep an ostomy supply backpack or travel bag. Keep this bag stocked with a few ostomy bags, a pair of scissors, skin cream, a couple of towels, gauze, paper towels, small plastic disposable bag or trash bag, and an extra pair of clothing for your child.

2) DO create a stoma cut out template: Getting the correct size of the cut out of the stoma bag is important. Too big of the cut out hole of the stoma bag will result in exposure of the surrounding abdominal skin to stool, which then will lead to skin irritation. Once you have established the correct size of the cut out hole in the stoma bag, save this stoma bag as a "master template". Use the template to cutting all future stoma bag cut outs. Also, have a few prepared cut outs handy, so that you don't have to worry about cutting out the hole in the bag when you may be outside the home or in a hurry.

3) DO care for the sensitive skin around the stoma: Even when you take the best precautions, it is likely that the abdominal skin around the stoma can sometimes become irritated, either because of continuous exposure to the adhesive circular patch of the ostomy bag and/or exposure to stool. One natural remedy is to simply air out the stoma – leave it exposed to the atmosphere and let the skin breathe for a few minutes. This is no different than what you would do for a child when he

or she has a bad diaper rash. Of course, the option is viable mostly when you are at home vs outside the house. Just know that the stoma is not going to continuously secrete stool, so letting it air for a few minutes is usually not that risky of a proposition. Also, airing out the stoma for a couple of minutes before placing on a new ostomy bag also proves to be a good skin protection strategy in the long run.

4) DO protect the skin: Use skin protection creams to treat irritation of the abdomen around the stoma.

Resources:

a) Hollister and Convatec are two of the popular makes for ostomy supplies including ostomy bags.

b) Skin barrier sprays are available and are recommended to be used to protect the skin.

c) Skin care:

    i.   Recommend using A&D Ointment for daily use. Best to use after colostomy closure operation to use a small amount after each diaper change, so that it will act as a barrier on the skin.

    ii.   Recommend using Triple Paste ointment in case of severe rash.

d) Various odor eliminating sprays made by Hollister and Convatec are available. Spray inside the stoma bag or use a few drops to control odor.

e) Adhesive removers may be used as appropriate, so the skin around the stoma does not get pulled each time you remove an old ostomy bag.

f) Venting the bag regularly is also recommended to get the most life out of each bag.

F.
HELPFUL DO'S AND DON'TS FOR PARENTS / FAMILIES OF CHILDREN WITH ANORECTAL MALFORMATIONS

1. Don't blame yourself.
2. It's ok to be disheartened, but don't be discouraged.
3. Do focus on what you can do, not on what should have been.
4. Don't hesitate to ask for help from your trusted friends and family.
5. Don't forget to take care of yourselves too, while you are focused on taking care of your child.
6. If you have other small children, be proactive about how you can arrange to get help from friends or family to watch them at times when you will be busy for hours or days of intensive care management for your child.
7. Do take the time to research in and out of network costs involved, if you have private insurance. Investigate and consider a second insurance if the state that you live offers it and if it works for you. Better to do this earlier rather than later.
8. Don't hesitate to ask for simplified explanations of medical terms or for important care related information to be repeated.
9. Don't settle for average or mediocre care and treatment. Do your own research and find out what the "ideal" treatment is for your child.

10. Do trust, but verify that your child is getting appropriate and timely care. See roadmap and initial reading material included in the appendix.
11. Do interact and connect with other parents in a similar situation. The treatments may not be the same for your children, but tips and tricks to manage the condition can be learned and exchanged and a sense of companionship may be therapeutic on the long journey.
12. Do brace yourself for the long journey. Hope for the best, but be prepared to adjust and course correct as required.
13. Do enjoy each day with your baby and don't short change yourself of any activities or vacations you may have otherwise taken.
14. Journal, journal, journal... Keep a log of everything as your baby progresses. This will be very helpful in the long run.
15. Last but not least: Be a fearless and strong advocate for your child.

Made in the USA
Columbia, SC
02 August 2020